STATISTICAL THINKING IN EPIDEMIOLOGY

STATISTICAL THINKING IN EPIDEMIOLOGY

YU-KANG TU
MARK S. GILTHORPE

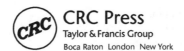

CRC Press
Taylor & Francis Group
Boca Raton London New York

CRC Press is an imprint of the
Taylor & Francis Group, an **informa** business
A CHAPMAN & HALL BOOK

CRC Press
Taylor & Francis Group
6000 Broken Sound Parkway NW, Suite 300
Boca Raton, FL 33487-2742

First issued in paperback 2019

© 2012 by Taylor & Francis Group, LLC
CRC Press is an imprint of Taylor & Francis Group, an Informa business

No claim to original U.S. Government works

ISBN-13: 978-1-4200-9991-1 (hbk)
ISBN-13: 978-0-367-38255-1 (pbk)

Visit the Taylor & Francis Web site at
http://www.taylorandfrancis.com

and the CRC Press Web site at
http://www.crcpress.com

Contents

Preface

Many books have been written on epidemiological methods. The main difference between them and this book is that we emphasise statistical thinking more than applications of specific statistical methods in epidemiological research, because we believe it is vital to appreciate context and for this to happen, one has to stop and reflect, rather than plough in. This book is therefore not a textbook for the statistical methods commonly used by biostatisticians and epidemiologists; instead, we assume readers have a basic understanding of generalised linear models, such as multiple regression and logistic regression. We do, however, discuss some basic methods in great detail, such as Pearson's correlation and the analysis of covariance, and we show that sometimes it requires a lot of careful thinking to use these simple methods correctly.

We use a few real examples, some of which remain controversial in epidemiological research, to demonstrate our statistical thinking. However, we by no means feel that our thinking is the only approach to the problems we highlight, which are chosen because we believe they have an appeal to general readers. Postgraduate students in biostatistics and epidemiology may use this book as a supplementary reading to standard texts on statistical or epidemiological methods. Lecturers of postgraduate courses may use this book (we hope) as a good example for teaching statistical thinking in epidemiological research. Experienced researchers may find our book both intellectually entertaining and challenging, as some issues discussed are still controversial. We try to show how our statistical thinking of specific research questions develops and eventually leads us to a set of solutions, but our thinking is inevitably framed by our training, knowledge, and experience. For instance, we believe vector geometry is a very useful tool for intuitive understanding of the basic concepts and nuances of linear models, but we acknowledge that not all our readers will agree with us as some may not find thinking geometrically at all intuitive or helpful. Therefore, we welcome feedback from our readers to broaden our vision and improve our thinking, hopefully giving rise to better solutions to those problems discussed in this book.

Our students, collaborators, and colleagues have been very helpful in sharpening and improving our thinking, and the following is an incomplete list of those we would wish to acknowledge and thank for their help in this regard: our colleagues in the Division of Biostatistics and the Division of Epidemiology at the University of Leeds; Professor George Ellison at the London Metropolitan University; Professor David Gunnell, Professor Jonathan Sterne and Dr. Kate Tilling at the University of Bristol; Professor Vibeke Baelum at Aarhus University, Denmark; Dr. Samuel Manda at the

Biostatistics Unit, Medical Research Council, South Africa; and Professor Kuo-Liong Chien at the National Taiwan University, Taiwan. Dr. Chris Metcalfe at the University of Bristol and Dr. Jim Lewsey at Glasgow University kindly acted as external reviewers for our book and gave many useful comments and suggestions. Nevertheless, we take full responsibility for any weakness and errors in our thinking in this book. We would also like to thank Sarah Morris and Rob Calver at Chapman & Hall for their patience with this project.

Part of this book was written when the first author (YKT) was on study leave in Taiwan supported by an international joint project grant from the Royal Society and the National Science Council in Taiwan. In the last 5 years, the first author has been supported by a UK Research Council Fellowship jointly housed by the School of Medicine (Division of Biostatistics) and the Leeds Dental Institute, having enjoyed a large degree of academic freedom in research supported by both the second author (head of the Division of Biostatistics) and Dr. Margaret Kellett (dean of the Leeds Dental Institute). Their generous support is greatly appreciated.

Finally, we would like to thank our wives, Jorin and Amy, and our daughters, Emma and Zarana, for their unconditional love and support.

1

Introduction

1.1 Uses of Statistics in Medicine and Epidemiology

Correlation and regression analyses are among the most commonly used statistical methods in biomedical research. Correlation tests the linear relationship between two (usually continuous) variables, and linear regression tests the relationship between one outcome variable (also known as the dependent variable) and one or more explanatory variables (also known as independent variables or covariates).

As powerful personal computers and graphical user-interface (GUI) statistical software packages have become available and readily affordable in the last decade, complex statistical methods such as multivariable regression become more and more frequently used in medicine and epidemiology, despite involving complex numerical calculations. For instance, to obtain the regression coefficients for a multiple linear regression model with five covariates, one needs to invert a 5×5 matrix, which is very complex and might take days to do by hand. With the power of computers, it now only takes a few seconds to perform these calculations, and all the information relevant (or irrelevant) to the research questions can be shown on the computer screen.

Unfortunately, whilst biomedical researchers may be able to follow instructions in the manuals accompanying the statistical software packages, they do not always have sufficient knowledge to choose the appropriate statistical methods and correctly interpret their results. Many biostatisticians have noticed that the misuses of statistical methods in clinical research are common and the quality of statistical reports in clinical journals needs to be improved (Altman 1991b, 1998, 2002; Andersen 1990). Besides, the increasing use of more advanced and complex statistical methods does not necessarily provide greater insight into the research questions and thereby obtain more reliable knowledge. On the contrary, careless use of these methods can sometimes generate confusing or even misleading results.

This book examines several common methodological and statistical problems in the use of correlation and regression in medical and epidemiological research: mathematical coupling, regression to the mean, collinearity, reversal paradox and statistical interaction. These problems are usually intertwined with each other. For instance, in the analysis of the relation between change and initial value, mathematical coupling and regression to the mean are almost synonymous; mathematical coupling between explanatory variables usually gives rise to collinearity; and product interaction terms and their component variables are mathematically coupled and raise concerns over collinearity. Since the discussions of these five problems pervade all areas of medical and epidemiological research, it is necessary to study these problems in a framework that focuses on specific research themes. Therefore, this book aims to examine the problems of mathematical coupling and regression to the mean in the analysis of change in pre-test/post-test study designs. The evidence on the foetal origins of adult diseases hypothesis, which sometimes suffers problems of the reversal paradox caused by the adjustment of current body size as confounders, is used to illustrate the potential problems in selecting variables for statistical adjustment and testing statistical interaction.

The overall aim of this book is to explore these statistical problems, to critically evaluate the existing proposed solutions to these problems, and to develop new tools to overcome them. One specific feature of this book is that, wherever applicable, vector geometry is used as a mathematical tool, in novel ways, to illustrate and further develop the concepts behind these statistical methods. The advantage of a geometrical approach over an analytical (algebraic) approach is that geometry can be more readily visualised and may be more intuitive to non-statisticians. Some common uses and misuses of correlation and regression analyses can be more intuitively understood by using geometrical illustrations than using traditional algebraic formula. Moreover, geometry will not only enhance our understanding of statistical problems, but will also generate new insights into old problems, thereby paving the way to provide guidance as to how to avoid statistical errors or even to suggest solutions.

1.2 Structure and Objectives of This Book

This book begins in Chapter 2 with a concise introduction to the concepts underlying the uses of vector geometry in linear models. Although vector geometry has been shown to be a great tool for understanding statistical methods based on ordinary least squares techniques, discussions of vector geometry are, however, scattered in the statistical literature only, and none appear in the clinical literature. So the objective of Chapter 2 is to bring together the various elementary results in vector geometry and establish a set of basic geometric tools that will be utilised throughout this book.

In Chapter 3, we introduce the concepts of directed acyclic graphs (DAGs). DAGs have become popular in epidemiological research in recent years as it provides a very useful tool for identifying potential confounders. It is very similar to path diagram for structural equation modelling, which is widely used in social sciences research for testing causal models.

Chapter 4 reviews a controversy in analysing the relation between change and initial value caused by mathematical coupling and regression to the mean. In the analyses of pre-test/post-test study design, it is difficult to distinguish between regression to the mean and mathematical coupling, and this difficulty has given rise to confusion amongst some statisticians surrounding how to solve the problem. The objectives of Chapter 4 are to demonstrate the inadequacy of current practice in clinical research, to correct a misconception amongst some statisticians and to review various statistical methods proposed to test the relation between change and initial value.

Chapter 5 explores the differences in statistical power and effect estimations between several statistical methods to analyse changes in the pre-test/ post-test study design for both randomised and non-randomised studies. The objectives of Chapter 5 are first to illustrate, using vector geometry, the controversy about the adjustment of initial values, known as *Lord's paradox*, and to explain why and when this paradox arises. This is particularly pertinent to epidemiology since Lord's paradox arises where proper randomisation is not always feasible—as within most epidemiological research. Vector geometry and simulations are then used to show that the prevalent concept that analysis of covariance (ANCOVA) *always* has greater statistical power than other univariate methods is not strictly correct; only when sample sizes are large and/or the correlation between pre-test and post-test values are moderate or high does ANCOVA have greater statistical power than other univariate and multivariate methods.

The objective of Chapter 6 is to demonstrate that vector geometry can give new insights into the problems of collinearity and the detection of these problems in epidemiological research. Collinearity is especially important in observational studies, where the underlying premise of statistical adjustment in regression models is to control simultaneously for correlations amongst covariates and their correlations with the outcome. Vector geometry can elegantly show why principal component analysis, a commonly recommended solution to collinearity, is not always desirable.

Chapter 7 discusses the problem of the reversal paradox, which is perhaps better known in epidemiology as *Simpson's paradox* within categorical variable analysis. In regression analysis, or analysis of covariance, this phenomenon is known as Lord's paradox, and in general linear modelling, a widely discussed statistical paradox known as *suppression* or *enhancement* is another manifestation of the reversal paradox. The objectives of Chapter 7 are to use the foetal origins of adult diseases hypothesis as an example to show how and why the adjustment of current body size measures, such as current body weight, can give rise to the reversal paradox in multiple linear regression. Vector geometry is used to illustrate the reversal paradox and question an alternative interpretation often proffered, namely, that catch-up growth has a greater impact than birth weight on health in later life. Computer simulations and evidence from empirical studies are then used to show that the negative relationships between birth weight and blood pressure are strengthened and positive relationships between birth weight and blood pressure are attenuated or even reversed after adjusting for one or more current body sizes.

Chapter 8 examines the role of statistical interaction within regression analyses by revisiting the four-model principle proposed in the foetal origins hypothesis literature. The objectives of this chapter are first to show that when three continuous variables, such as blood pressure, birth weight and current body weight, follow multivariate normality, the expected value of the partial regression coefficient for the product interaction term in the multiple regression model is zero. Computer simulations are used to show that categorising birth weight and/or current body weight, a common practice in epidemiological studies on the foetal origins hypothesis (and many epidemiological studies in general), gives rise to spurious interaction effects and can therefore potentially lead to seriously misleading conclusions.

Chapter 9 reviews the recent advances in identifying critical growth phases for health outcomes in later life. In recent years, some researchers' interests have shifted from birth size to the growth in body size during early childhood. In Chapter 9 we provide a concise introduction to those methods for identifying the critical growth phases and use a publicly available data set to illustrate and compare results. This chapter shows that whilst different statistical methods have been proposed to test the same hypothesis, the differences in those approaches seem to indicate that researchers may have different versions of the same hypothesis in mind. As statistical thinking is guided by the research hypothesis, differences in theorising and framing the research questions will inevitably lead to different thinkings.

After discussing the pros and cons of the proposed methods for identifying the critical growth phases within Chapter 9, we propose a new approach in Chapter 10 that uses partial least squares (PLS). PLS is widely used in chemometrics and bioinformatics, though it is rarely used in medical and epidemiological research. One apparent advantage of PLS is that it can deal with perfect collinearity that can arise due to the mathematical relationships amongst covariates. In Chapter 10 we use the same data set as in Chapter 9 to illustrate how PLS can be applied to lifecourse research.

Most of the data sets used in this book have been drawn from published literature that are easily obtainable. One data set was kindly made available by Dr. Lars Laurell.

1.3 Nomenclature in This Book

Italic capital letters (X) denote variables without measurement error.

Italic lower-case letters (x) denote observed variables measured with error.

Bold lower-case letters (**x**) denote vectors.

Bold capital letters (**X**) denote matrices.

Capital letters (X) with subscripts denote components of variables or vectors.

Subscripts of variables usually represent repeated observations on the same variables, though they may also represent levels within a multilevel framework.

1.4 Glossary

Due to our backgrounds and a number of extensive collaborations with dental researchers, we sometimes use examples from the dental literature to illustrate methodological problems. Consequently, non-dental readers might not be familiar with some of the terminology that frequently appears in some chapters. This section provides a non-technical explanation and illustration (Figure 1.1a and b) of the dental terminology.

Clinical attachment level (CAL): The distance between the cemento-enamel junction and the bottom of periodontal pocket. It is not common to measure CAL directly using a periodontal probe; instead, CAL is usually the sum of gingival recession (GR) and probing pocket depth (PPD).

Enamel matrix proteins derivatives (EMD): Extracts from developing teeth in young pigs; these mixtures of proteins are believed to be able to promote regeneration of lost periodontal tissue. A syringe is used to release EMD into periodontal infrabony defects.

Gingival recession (GR): The distance between the cemento-enamel junctions and the gingival margin. In a healthy condition, the level of gingival margin (i.e., gums) is assumed to be level with the cemento-enamel junction and, therefore, GR is zero. However, due to external trauma, periodontal diseases or aging, the gingival margins may recede; that is, move in the direction of the root apex, and GR

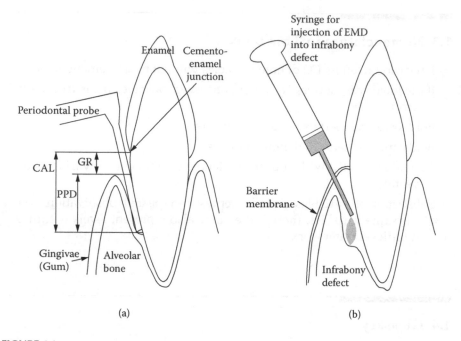

(a)   (b)

FIGURE 1.1
Illustration of the glossary. (a) Measurement of periodontal pocket depths; (b) application EMD in periodontal surgery.

is positive. In some circumstances, the gingivae (i.e., gums) might cover part of the crown of the tooth and the cemento-enamel junction becomes invisible, in which case GR is negative.

Guided tissue regeneration (GTR): A surgical procedure to regenerate lost periodontal tissue, especially in periodontal infrabony defects and furcation involvement in molars. A barrier membrane is placed around the tooth to cover the defect in order to allow progenitor cells from alveolar bone and/or periodontal membrane to repopulate on the root surface.

Probing (pocket) depth (PD): The distance between the gingival margin and the bottom of the periodontal pockets. Both PD and GR are usually measured with a periodontal probe with markings in millimetres. In this book, probing pocket depth, probing depth or pocket depth are all equivalent and used interchangeably.

2

Vector Geometry of Linear
Models for Epidemiologists

2.1 Introduction

Vector geometry was first used in 1915 (Fisher 1915) by the great statistician Sir Ronald Fisher to address the problem of deriving the statistical distribution of the Pearson product–moment correlation coefficient. Fisher used his great geometric imagination to demonstrate that the correlation between two variables is the cosine function of the angle between two vectors in an n-dimensional space. However, as most statisticians do not have the same great geometrical insights as Fisher did, and most statisticians consider an algebraic approach more mathematically rigorous, the geometric approach has not thus far received as much attention as it perhaps deserves (Herr 1980). Nevertheless, some teachers of statistics have found a geometric approach to be more intuitive for people without a mathematical background and a very useful tool to develop the understanding of linear regression analyses. A few statistical textbooks (Saville and Wood 1991, 1996; Wickens 1995; Carroll et al. 1997) are written using mainly vector geometry, and some textbooks of statistics or econometrics on linear statistical models (Wonnacott and Wonnacott 1979, 1981; Fox 1997; Draper and Smith 1998) have chapters on vector geometry. However, vector geometry seems to have been used rarely to illustrate or explore specific methodological problems within biomedical research.

The aim of this chapter is to provide an introduction to the various concepts of vector geometry within correlation and regression analyses. Vector geometry, as a mathematical tool, will be consistently and extensively explored in later chapters.

2.2 Basic Concepts of Vector Geometry in Statistics

The scatter plot, one of the most commonly used graphs to display the relationship between two continuous variables, can be viewed as a form of geometry. In the scatter plot for two random variables, X and Y, each with n independent observations $(X_1 \ldots X_n)$ and $(Y_1 \ldots Y_n)$, there will be n points in *two*-dimensional space (i.e., on a plane). This is known as *variable space* geometry. The axes represent the variables X and Y, and the points are the observations made on each subject. In contrast, instead of using variables as axes, the same data can be displayed in what is termed *subject space* by using subjects as the axes; the variables X and Y are then two points in n-dimensional space. By drawing an arrow from the origin to each point, X and Y become two vectors with coordinates $(X_1 \ldots X_n)$ and $(Y_1 \ldots Y_n)$ in n-dimensional space (Wickens 1995; Fox 1997). Although it is impossible to visualise n-dimensional space, only a plane is required to visualise the relative relationship between the vectors representing X and Y in n-dimensional space by projecting onto a plane and effectively dropping the original axes. In general, the number of dimensions needed to draw the graph in subject space is no greater than the number of variables (Wickens 1995).

We use a numerical example to illustrate the difference in data presentation between variable-space (scatter plot) geometry and subject-space (vector) geometry. Suppose two men, Mr A and Mr B, have their body size measured: the heights of A and B are 180 cm and 170 cm, respectively, and their weights are 90 kg and 60 kg, respectively. When the data are presented in a scatter plot (i.e., variable-space), subjects A and B are two points in a two-dimensional plot, and the axes are *Height* and *Weight* (Figure 2.1a). When the same data are presented in vector geometry (subject space), *Height* and *Weight* become two vectors in a two-dimensional space, and subjects A and B are the axes (Figure 2.1b).

In Figure 2.1b, the two variables *Height* and *Weight* are presented in their raw data format. However, in general, it is very useful to represent the

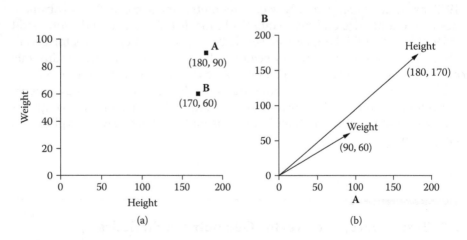

FIGURE 2.1
Illustrations of variable-space (a) and subject-space (b) geometry.

original variables as scaled vectors such that, for x, for instance, each X_i value is transformed so that the length of the new vector, denoted $\|x\|$, is equal to the standard deviation (SD) of the original data by using the formula

$$X_i^{new} = \frac{\left[X_i^{old} - \left(\sum_{i=1}^{n} X_i^{old} / n \right) \right]}{\sqrt{n-1}}. \tag{2.1}$$

Other variables, such as y and z, are similarly transformed to yield the vectors y and z. An immediate advantage is that the Pearson correlation coefficient between X and Y is the cosine of the angle between vectors x and y. For instance, when the correlation between X and Y is zero, the angle between x and y is 90° (or $\pi/2$ radians), and these two vectors are therefore said to be orthogonal; that is, perpendicular (denoted $x \perp y$). Similarly, when the correlation between X and Y is 0.5, the angle between x and y is 60° ($\pi/3$ radians).

Another advantage of representing these variables as scaled vectors is that the number of dimensions needed for presentation of regression analysis is reduced by one. For instance, when y is regressed on x, there are three variables in the equation: y, x and the *intercept*. The intercept is a vector with its entire elements being 1; that is, i is a column vector = $[1 \ldots 1]$. After transformation using Equation 2.1, i becomes zero and hence redundant. Therefore, we need only two dimensions to draw the graph of two-variable regression in subject space.

2.3 Correlation and Simple Regression in Vector Geometry

Whilst the correlation coefficient between two scaled variables is their angle between the vectors, the regression coefficient is the orthogonal (perpendicular) projection of the outcome variable vector on the covariate vector. For instance, for two variables x and y, their correlation coefficient $r_{xy} = \cos(\theta_{xy})$, where θ_{xy} is the angle between vectors x and y (Figure 2.2), and the regression coefficient b_x is the length of projection of y on x divided by the length of x ($\|x\|$); that is, $\cos(\theta_{xy})$ multiplied by the ratio of length of y ($\|y\|$) divided by $\|x\|$ (Figure 2.2). All vectors are presented as a line with an arrow, where the length of the line is the length of the vector and the arrow is the direction of the vector in vector space; the size of the arrow is irrelevant to the length of the vector.

Suppose variable y is the measurement of body weight in kilograms for five people: y = {60, 65, 70, 75, 80}. To present y as a vector, we use Equation 2.1 to rescale y to obtain y = {−5, −2.5, 0, 2.5, 5}. The length of vector y is defined as

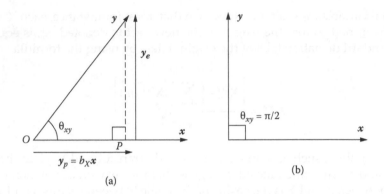

FIGURE 2.2

(a) A vector illustration of correlation and simple regression: variable Y (represented by vector y) correlated with/regressed on variable X (represented by vector x), and (b) illustration that if variables Y and X are uncorrelated, their corresponding vectors are orthogonal. (a) The correlation between variables Y and X (r_{XY}) is the cosine of θ_{xy}, the angle between vectors x and y; the projection of y on x (denoted y_p) has length $\|y\|.\cos(\theta_{xy})$. Vector y_p lies in the same direction as vector x and may therefore be expressed as a multiple of x: $y_p = b_X x$, where $b_X = (\|y\|/\|x\|)\cos(\theta_{xy})$ is the simple regression coefficient for X when Y is regressed on X. The residual vector y_e is derived by $y - y_p$ (and for illustration the origin of y_e is drawn at the tip of y_p). (b) If $\theta_{xy} = 90°$ ($\pi/2$ radians), then x and y are orthogonal (denoted $x \perp y$), and the correlation between X and Y is zero: $\rho_{XY} = \cos(90°) = \cos(\pi/2) = 0$. Consequently, the regression coefficient for y regressed on x is also zero.

$$\|y\| = \sqrt{(-5)^2 + (-2.5)^2 + (0)^2 + (2.5)^2 + (5)^2} = 7.9,$$

and this is also the standard deviation of y. Suppose another variable x is the measurement of body height in centimetres for these five people: $x = \{160, 160, 170, 180, 180\}$. To present x as a vector, we use Equation 2.1 to rescale x to obtain $x = \{-5, -5, 0, 5, 5\}$. The length of vector x is defined as

$$\|x\| = \sqrt{(-5)^2 + (-5)^2 + (0)^2 + (5)^2 + (5)^2} = 10,$$

and this is the SD of x. After rescaling the original variables, the length of their vectors is always equal to the SD of the original variables.

In mathematics, vectors are usually written as a column vector, for example, $y = \{-5, -2.5, 0, 2.5, 5\}$ is usually written as

$$y = \begin{bmatrix} -5 \\ -2.5 \\ 0 \\ 2.5 \\ 5 \end{bmatrix},$$

and the transpose of **y**, denoted $\mathbf{y}^T$, is a row vector: $\mathbf{y}^T = [-5 \quad -2.5 \quad 0 \quad 2.5 \quad 5]$.

One important advantage of presenting variables as vectors is that the angle between two vectors has an important statistical property: the cosine of the angle between vectors **y** and **x** is the correlation coefficient between *weight* and *height*.

Another important statistical property is the orthogonal projection of **y** on **x**. In Figure 2.2, a line denoted *L* (the dashed line) is drawn from the tip of **y** to **x**, making the angle between *L* and **x** 90°, and the point *P*, where *L* and **x** meet, determines the length of the projection of **y** on **x**. Elementary trigonometry shows that *L* has the shortest length amongst all possible lines drawn from the tip of **y** to any point on **x**. It is important to note that the length from *O* (the origin of **y** and **x**) to *P* (on **x**), denoted $\overline{OP}$, divided by the length of **x**, will be the regression coefficient for *Y* regressed on *X*. Mathematically, the length of $\overline{OP}$ is given as

$$\|\overline{OP}\| = \frac{\mathbf{y}^T\mathbf{x}}{\|\mathbf{x}\|} = \frac{\left((-5*-5)+(-2.5*-5)+(0*0)+(2.5*5)+(5*5)\right)}{10} = 7.5,$$

where $\mathbf{y}^T\mathbf{x}$ denoted the inner product of vectors **y** and **x** (which is the sum of the products of the first element of **y** multiplied by the first element of **x** and similarly for all subsequent *i*th elements of **y** and **x**). Thus, the orthogonal projection of **y** on **x** equates to the inner product of **y** and **x** divided by the length of **x**. The regression coefficient is therefore 7.5/10 = 0.75. Recall that when *y* is regressed on *x*, the regression coefficient for *x* is given as

$$b_x = \frac{Cov(y,x)}{Var(x)},$$

where $Cov(y,x)$ is the covariance of *y* and *x*, and $Var(x)$ is the variance of *x*. It becomes clear that the inner product of vectors **y** and **x** is the covariance of variables *y* and *x*, and the variance of *x* is the square of the length of vector **x**.

2.4 Linear Multiple Regression in Vector Geometry

To regress the variable *y* on the two variables *x* and *z* is equivalent, within vector geometry, to finding the orthogonal projection of the vector **y** on the plane spanned by the vectors **x** and **z** and then to use the parallelogram rule to find the contributing proportions of **x** and **z** that yield the projected vector $\mathbf{y}_p$. For instance, we denote the regression equation for these variables as $y = b_x x + b_z z$, where b_x and b_z are partial regression coefficients.

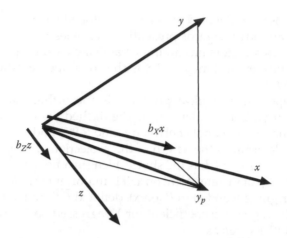

FIGURE 2.3
Vector illustration of multiple regression: variable *Y* (represented by vector *y*) regressed (simultaneously) on variable *X* (represented by vector *x*) and variable *Z* (represented by vector *z*). (a) The projection of *y* ($\mathbf{y}_p$) onto the plane spanned by *x* and *z* comprises the appropriate proportions of the vectors *x* and *z*; the proportion of vector *x* is b_X, and the proportion of *z* is b_Z. These proportions are derived by means of the parallelogram rule: $\mathbf{y}_p$ is projected parallel to *z* onto *x* to obtain the proportion b_X of *x*, and $\mathbf{y}_p$ is projected parallel to *x* onto *z* to obtain the proportion b_Z of *z*.

Using vector geometry, $\mathbf{y}_p = b_X\mathbf{x} + b_Z\mathbf{z}$, where b_X and b_Z are the proportions (projection weights) of the vectors **x** and **z** that make up $\mathbf{y}_p$ (Figure 2.3).

2.5 Significance Testing of Correlation and Simple Regression in Vector Geometry

To test whether or not the correlation between *x* and $y(r_{xy})$ and regression coefficient b_x when *y* is regressed on *x* is statistically significant at a specified threshold probability from a geometric perspective is to test whether or not the angle θ_{xy} between vector **x** and **y** is smaller than a specified threshold angle. In Figure 2.2, it is shown that *vector y can* be decomposed as two perpendicular vectors $\mathbf{y}_p$ and $\mathbf{y}_e$. Vector $\mathbf{y}_p$ is in the same direction as **x**, and $\mathbf{y}_e$ is perpendicular (orthogonal) to $\mathbf{y}_p$ and **x**. From trigonometry, the smaller θ_{xy}, the greater the value of $\cos(\theta_{xy})$ and the greater the ratio of $\|\mathbf{y}_p\|/\|\mathbf{y}_e\|$, where $\|\mathbf{y}_e\|$ and $\|\mathbf{y}_p\|$ are the lengths of vectors $\mathbf{y}_e$ and $\mathbf{y}_p$. The *F* ratio test for the correlation r_{xy} or regression coefficient b_x is thus given as (Wickens 1995; Saville and Wood 1996)

$$F_{(p,n-p-1)} = \frac{\|\mathbf{y}_p\|^2/p}{\|\mathbf{y}_e\|^2/(n-p-1)}, \tag{2.2}$$

where p is the number of degrees of freedom of all covariates; that is, $p = 1$ in this example, and n is the sample size. Therefore, the formula can be rearranged for this specific example as

$$F_{(1,n-2)} = \frac{\|\mathbf{y}_p\|^2 (n-2)}{\|\mathbf{y}_e\|^2}. \tag{2.3}$$

It is noted that the concept of degrees of freedom, which many non-statisticians find hard to comprehend, can be understood via vector geometry. The multiplier, $(n-2)$, in the numerator of the F-test is the degrees of freedom of vector $\mathbf{y}_e$, and $\|\mathbf{y}_e\|^2$ is the *sum of squared errors*. For variables x and y with sample size n, the original vector space is n dimensions. As x and y are rescaled to reduce one dimension, vectors $\mathbf{x}$ and $\mathbf{y}$ are now in $n-1$ dimensional space. As shown in Figure 2.2, vector $\mathbf{y}$ is decomposed as $\mathbf{y}_p$ and $\mathbf{y}_e$. However, for any vector $\mathbf{y}_e'$, which has the same length of $\mathbf{y}_e$ but in a different direction from $\mathbf{y}_e$ (e.g., out of the plane in our three-dimensional representation), the sum of $\mathbf{y}_e'$ and $\mathbf{y}_p$ will create a vector $\mathbf{y}'$, and the angle between any $\mathbf{y}'$ and $\mathbf{x}$ will be the *same* as the angle θ_{xy} between $\mathbf{y}$ and $\mathbf{x}$. The three-dimensional projection of the subspace of $\mathbf{y}'$ is, in fact, a cone with its tip at the origin and its central axis along $\mathbf{x}$ (Figure 2.4). Therefore, any pair of vectors $\mathbf{y}'$ and $\mathbf{x}$ will have the same correlation and regression coefficient. Except for the direction of x, all the other dimensions perpendicular to $\mathbf{x}$ will be permissible for $\mathbf{y}_e'$. As a result, the possible number of dimensions for any $\mathbf{y}_e'$ is the total number of dimension (now $n-1$ because of the scaling) less the dimension of x; that is, $(n-1)-1 = n-2$, which is thus the number of *degrees of freedom* for $\mathbf{y}_e'$ (Wickens 1995; Fox 1997) in this instance.

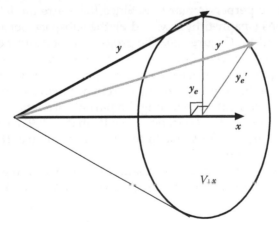

FIGURE 2.4
Geometrical illustration of degrees of freedom of the error vector. As x and y are scaled vectors in an $n-1$ dimensional space, the permissible subspace ($V_{\perp x}$) for any vector orthogonal to x is $n-2$ dimensional.

From Equation 2.3, it is obvious that when the correlation between x and y is fixed; that is, the angle between vectors $\mathbf{x}$ and $\mathbf{y}$ is constant, the greater the sample size, the greater the F-value (and therefore, the smaller the P-value). Therefore, to increase the statistical power of a study, one has either to increase its sample size or the effect size (for example, the correlation coefficient). It is well known that the F-values of $F(1,n)$ are equal to squares of the t-values of $t(n)$, so these two tests will yield the same results (Saville and Wood 1996; Draper and Smith 1998). Commercial statistical packages usually report the F-values in analysis of variance (ANOVA) tables for regression analyses, and the t-values in tables for regression coefficients; these are effectively synonymous.

2.6 Significance Testing of Multiple Regression in Vector Geometry

Testing the regression coefficient b_x for x when y is regressed on x and z is slightly more complex. The significance test of b_x in multiple regression is to test the independent contribution of x to the explained variance of y. The P-value for partial regression coefficients obtained when controlling for other covariates is derived, within vector geometry, from the projection of the covariate vectors whose coefficient is being tested and the outcome vector onto the subspace that is perpendicular to all remaining covariates (Wickens 1995). For instance, when regressing y on both x and z, the P-value for the partial regression coefficient for x is derived from the projection of $\mathbf{x}$ and $\mathbf{y}$ onto the subspace perpendicular to $\mathbf{z}$. Since the entire model space is only three dimensions (spanned by $\mathbf{x}$, $\mathbf{y}$, and $\mathbf{z}$), the subspace perpendicular to $\mathbf{z}$ is a plane denoted $V_{\perp z}$ (Figure 2.5). The projections of y and x on $V_{\perp z}$ are vectors $\mathbf{y}_{\perp z}$ and $\mathbf{x}_{\perp z}$, respectively. The strength of the association between y and x, whilst adjusting for z, is evaluated by assessing the angle between $\mathbf{y}_{\perp z}$ and $\mathbf{x}_{\perp z}$ (i.e. the correlation between $\mathbf{y}_{\perp z}$ and $\mathbf{x}_{\perp z}$). From a statistical regression model viewpoint, this is equivalent to testing the partial correlation between y and x after adjustment for z, $r_{xy.z}$ (Wickens 1995; Pedhazur 1997). From a geometric perspective, this is equivalent to testing the angle (i.e. the correlation) between vectors $\mathbf{y}_{\perp z}$ and $\mathbf{x}_{\perp z}$.

The F-ratio test for the partial correlation $r_{xy.z}$ or partial regression coefficient b_x whilst y is regressed on x and z is given as (Wickens 1995)

$$F_{(p,n-p-q-1)} = \frac{\|\mathbf{y}_{x\perp z}\|^2/p}{\|\mathbf{y}_e\|^2/(n-p-q-1)}, \qquad (2.4)$$

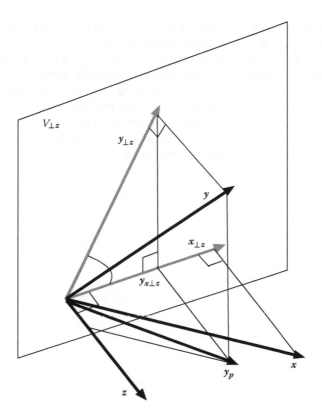

FIGURE 2.5
Vector illustration of significance testing in multiple regression. To test the partial regression coefficient of X (b_X), when Y is regressed on X whilst also adjusting for Z, is to test, within vector geometry, the relation between the projections onto the subspace perpendicular to z ($V_{\perp z}$) of y ($\mathbf{y}_{\perp z}$) and x ($\mathbf{x}_{\perp z}$).

where $\mathbf{y}_{x \perp z}$ is the projection of $\mathbf{y}_{\perp z}$ on $x_{\perp z}$ (which is equivalent to the projection of $\mathbf{y}$ on $\mathbf{x}_{\perp z}$), p is the degrees of freedom of x (i.e., $p = 1$ in this example), q is the degrees of freedom of z (i.e., $q = 1$), and n is the sample size.

2.7 Summary

In this chapter it is shown how statistical methods for the relationships between variables, such as correlation and regression analyses, can be understood as relationships amongst vectors in n-dimensional space. Commonly used test statistics, such as t-test and F-test, used in correlation and regression,

can be visualised geometrically. Although the figures of vectors representing multiple regression may look a little complex for beginners, the idea of
vector geometry is straightforward and intuitive: the correlation between
two variables is expressed as the angle between their corresponding vectors,
and regressing variable y on x and z simultaneously is to find the perpendicular projection of **y** on the **x-z** plane. The mathematical details, such as
how the projected vector is obtained, do not need to concern us here, as it is
only the conceptual understanding that is most useful for our comprehen-
sion of advanced issues discussed in later chapters.

3

Path Diagrams and Directed Acyclic Graphs

3.1 Introduction

Regression analysis is probably the most commonly used statistical method in medical and epidemiological research. Technically, all regression models, such as multiple linear regression for a continuous outcome, logistic regression for a binary outcome, or Poisson regression for counts, are within the family of generalised linear models (GLMs). For example, the regression model for a continuous Y regressed on p covariates is given as

$$y = b_0 + b_1 x_1 + b_2 x_2 + \ldots + b_p x_P + e. \tag{3.1}$$

Equation 3.1 provides the mathematical relationship between y and the p xs, though many researchers might also believe that this equation describes some biological relationship between y and the xs. An important task for epidemiologists is to infer the causal relation between y and just *one* x (because others are generally confounders). However, even if we accept that Equation 3.1 may represent a certain causal relation between y and the xs, it does not indicate what the relationships are amongst the xs. Many non-statisticians do not know how the regression coefficients (b_0 to b_p) are calculated and have little idea as to how the relationships amongst the covariates are treated within a regression analysis. For most users of statistics, the latter is crucial to the proper interpretation of regression models. In this chapter we will introduce the path diagram, which is commonly adopted in the structural equation modelling literature as a conceptual tool for understanding causal relationships amongst variables within regression models.

3.1 Path Diagrams

Structural equation modelling (SEM) can be considered a general theoretical framework for all univariate and multivariate linear statistical models; that is, correlation, linear regression, analysis of variance, multivariate analysis of variance, canonical correlation, and factor analysis (Bollen 1989; Loehlin 2004; Kline 2005). The statistical theory of SEM is complex, and the corresponding equations are usually written using matrix algebra. An alternative way for non-statisticians to appreciate the concepts of SEM is through understanding the path diagrams of the corresponding statistical models. Indeed, some software packages for structural equation modelling, such as AMOS (Amos Developmental Corporation, Spring House, PA), EQS (Multivariate Software, Encino, CA) and LISREL (Scientific Software International, Lincolnwood, IL), provide a graphical interface allowing users to draw path diagrams for their models on the computer screen, and the software then interprets this and performs the analyses specified in the path diagrams.

3.1.1 The Path Diagram for Simple Linear Regression

To illustrate what a path diagram is, we begin with the well-known example of a simple linear regression model with one outcome variable (known as the dependent variable) and one explanatory variable (known as the independent variable or covariate). Figure 3.1 is the path diagram for a simple linear regression model given as

$$y = b_0 + b_1 x + e, \tag{3.2}$$

where y is the outcome variable, x the explanatory variable, e the residual error term, b_0 the intercept, and b_1 the regression coefficient for x. The

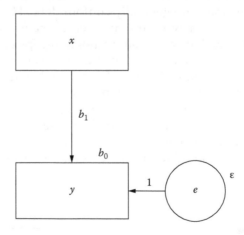

FIGURE 3.1
Path diagram of simple linear regression in Equation 3.1. For endogenous (dependent) variable y, the intercept b_0 is estimated. The regression coefficient b_1 in the path diagram is equivalent to the regression coefficient b_1 in Equation 3.1. For the residual error e, its mean is fixed to zero but its variance (ε) is estimated. The regression coefficient for e is always fixed to unity.

standard interpretation of Equation 3.2 is that when x is zero, y is b_0, and when x increases by one unit, y is expected to increase by the amount of b_1. The residual error term is the difference between the observed values of the outcome and the predicted (linear model) values of the outcome. In path diagrams, observed variables such as x and y are within squares, whereas latent (i.e., not directly measured and to be estimated in the model) variables such as residual errors (e in Equation 3.2) are within circles. An arrow from variable x to variable y in a path diagram means that x affects y in the specified statistical model, but y does not affect x. In contrast, a double arrow connecting x and y means that these two variables are correlated without specific causal directions. For instance, suppose x is children's age, and y is their body height. It is reasonable to draw an arrow from x to y as age causally determines body height. On the other hand, when x is body height and y is body weight, it is sensible to draw a double arrow because both variables are determined by other factors such as age. When there is no arrowed line (single or double) between x and y, this means that x and y are assumed to be causally independent; that is, the underlying population correlation between them is assumed to be zero in the specified model. In the linear regression model, x and e are assumed to be uncorrelated, which is one of the assumptions behind regression analysis: that is, explanatory variables and residual errors are independent. The arrow from one variable to another is called a *path* in the diagram. In Figure 3.1, there are two paths that specify the relationships amongst the variables in the model: one from x to y, and another from e to y. As a result, two parameters associated with those two paths may be estimated. The parameter for the path from x to y is b_1, which is unknown but can be estimated, whereas the parameter for the path from e to y is fixed to be 1. Thus, only one free (i.e., not already known or not fixed to certain value) parameter for the relationship between x and y requires estimation.

3.1.1.1 Regression Weights, Path Coefficients and Factor Loadings

In linear regression, b_1 is usually called the *regression coefficient*, but in structural equation models the parameters for the paths are sometimes called *path coefficients* or *factor loadings*. Despite the confusing jargon, all these terms can be interpreted as regression coefficients; here we simply call them regression coefficients. One exception is when a double arrow connects two variables (not in Figure 3.1), in which case the estimated path coefficient is the covariance between the two variables.

3.1.1.2 Exogenous and Endogenous Variables

In a path diagram such as Figure 3.1, variables like x are known as *exogenous variables* because there is no arrow from other variables in the model directed toward them. In contrast, variables like y are known as *endogenous variables* because there is at least one arrow from other variables in the model (x in this instance) directed toward it. Endogenous variables are accompanied by residual errors, such as e in our model, because it is unlikely that the variations in y can be completely explained by x. Structural equation modelling estimates the means and variances for exogenous variables whilst estimating the intercepts for the endogenous variables. This is because the variances of endogenous variables are derived from exogenous variables and associated residual errors. For example, in the linear regression given as Equation 3.2, the intercept for y will be estimated and is equivalent to b_0. Both the mean and variance of x will be estimated, though they are not explicitly expressed in Equation 3.2. The mean of the residual errors e is fixed to zero (as it is in regression analysis), and the path coefficient from it to the associated endogenous variable is fixed to be 1 (as it is in Equation 3.2). Therefore, the only parameter to be estimated is its variance. The mean and variance of y can then be derived from Equation 3.2. Note that observed and unobserved variables can be exogenous or endogenous variables.

3.1.2 The Path Diagram for Multiple Linear Regression

Multiple linear regression tests the relationship between one outcome variable, y, and more than one explanatory variable, $x_1, x_2, ..., x_p$. Figure 3.2 is the path diagram for a multiple linear regression with three explanatory variables denoted:

$$y = b_0 + b_1 x_1 + b_2 x_2 + b_3 x_3 + e, \tag{3.3}$$

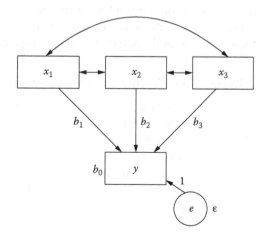

FIGURE 3.2
The path diagram for multiple regression in Equation 3.2. For endogenous (dependent) variable y, the intercept b_0 is estimated. The three regression coefficients (b_1, b_2 and b_3) in the path diagram are equivalent to those in Equation 3.2. For the residual error e, its mean is fixed to zero but its variance (ε) is estimated. The regression coefficient for e is always fixed to unity.

where y is the outcome variable, x_1 to x_3 are the explanatory variables, e is the residual error term, b_0 is the intercept, and b_1 to b_3 are the regression coefficients for x_1 to x_3, respectively. The standard interpretation of Equation 3.3 is that when x_1 to x_3 is zero, y is b_0, and when x_1 increases by one unit and x_2 and x_3 are held constant, y is expected to increase by the amount of b_1.

In Figure 3.2, the three paths from each of the three explanatory variables to y are equivalent to the regression coefficients given by Equation 3.3, and the interpretation of these paths is the same as that for the regression coefficients. Note that there are three double arrows in Figure 3.2 that connect x_1, x_2 and x_3, representing the covariance amongst the three explanatory variables (whose means and variances will also be estimated). This indicates that the relationship between y and each x is determined whilst also taking into account the correlations amongst the three explanatory variables. Note that when multiple regression analysis is undertaken using standard software packages, the explanatory variables are always assumed to be correlated, whether or not subsequent interpretation of the regression coefficients acknowledges this.

3.2 Directed Acyclic Graphs

One limitation of classical SEM analysis is that the manifest (observed) variables for endogenous variables have to be continuous variables (no such limitation for exogenous variables). Recent advances in SEM theory and software development have overcome this by implementing new estimation procedures. For instance, some SEM software, such as Mplus, allows for the variable y in Equation 3.3 and Figure 3.2 to be binary or ordinal. As many outcome variables in epidemiology are binary or counts, these new developments make SEM a useful tool for causal modelling in epidemiology. In fact, directed acyclic graphs (DAGs), which have been known to epidemiologists for nearly two decades but have received great attention in the last few years in particular, are very similar to path diagrams. DAGs have been mainly used by epidemiologists to identify confounders and potential biases in the estimation of causal relationships, though DAGs are path diagrams, except that, in SEM, two variables can be correlated without explicitly specifying the direction of their relationship. For instance, in Figure 3.3a, there is a double arrow between X and Z, and this means that we do not know the direction of their relationship. For SEM, this may not be a problem because this simply means that there is an unobserved or unmeasured variable U that is a causal parent of X and Z (Figure 3.3b). In DAGs, such a double arrow is not allowed, and therefore Figure 3.3a is not a DAG, though Figure 3.3b is. Also, error terms for endogenous variables in path diagrams are rarely explicitly

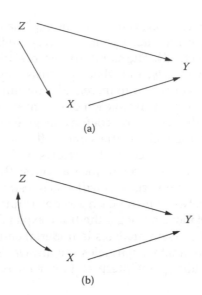

FIGURE 3.3
Illustrations of path diagram (a) and directed acyclic graph (b).

specified in DAGs, and this makes DAGs more like a qualitative version of path diagrams in SEM.

3.2.1 Identification of Confounders

Which variables should be adjusted for as confounders in a regression model has been a controversial issue within epidemiology (Weinberg 1993; Kirkwood and Sterne 2003; Jewell 2004), and only with the introduction of DAGs has this controversy been partially resolved (though not completely, as we will discuss later). According to DAGs theory, confounders are variables that are causally associated with the outcome and exposure but *not* on the causal path from the exposure to the outcome variable (Greenland et al. 1999; Pearl 2000; Glymour 2006; Glymour and Greenland 2008). For instance, variable Z is a confounder for the relation between the exposure X and the outcome Y in Figure 3.4a because there are arrows from Z to X and Y (i.e., they are causally associated), and Z is *not* on the causal path from X to Y. In contrast, Z is not a confounder for the relation between the exposure X and the outcome Y in Figure 3.4b because, although there are arrows from Z to Y and from X to Z (i.e., they are causally associated), Z is on the causal path from X to Y. Therefore, if we want to estimate the impact of X on Y, Z is a confounder and should be adjusted for according to Figure 3.4a, but Z is not a confounder according to Figure 3.4b.

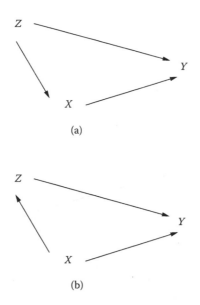

(a)

(b)

FIGURE 3.4
Illustrations of confounders in directed acyclic graphs. Z is a confounder for X in Figure 3.4a because it is causally related to the exposure X and the outcome Y, and Z is not on the causal path from X to Y. Z is not a confounder for X in Figure 3.4b because it is on the causal path from X to Y.

3.2.2 Backdoor Paths and Colliders

We may ask why Z is a confounder and should be adjusted for in Figure 3.4a and what would happen if Z is not adjusted for. Before we answer this question, we first look at Figure 3.5a, and the difference between Figure 3.4a and 3.5a is that there is no arrow from X to Y in Figure 3.5a. Suppose the arrow from Z to X and Y represents a positive association. When Z increases, we will observe that both X and Y increase. If we do not know that Z is behind the observed increases in X and Y, we may conclude that either X influences Y or vice versa, but actually, if we change the values of X (or Y), nothing would happen to Y (or X). Z is therefore a confounder for the relation between X and Y, and this can be identified by tracing the path from X to Y or Y to X. We first start with X and move in the reverse direction of the path directing to X (i.e., Z → X), and then we move in the same direction of the path going from Z to its causal children, such as Y. This is known as a *backdoor path* from X to Y via Z (Greenland et al. 1999; Pearl 2000; Glymour 2006; Glymour and Greenland 2008). When there are backdoor paths from the exposure to the outcome, the estimate of their causal relation is contaminated (in statistical jargon, *biased*).

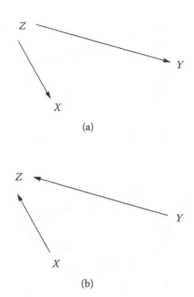

FIGURE 3.5

(a) Z is the common cause for X and Y; (b) both X and Y are causes of Z.

To block the backdoor paths, variables such as Z need to be adjusted for, and in epidemiological terminology, these variables are called *confounders*.

A related issue is to identify colliders in DAG. Consider Figure 3.5b. There are paths from X to Z and Y to Z; that is, changing either X or Y will give rise to change in Z, but changes in X will not cause changes in Y, and vice versa. However, if we adjust for Z when we regress Y on X (or X on Y), we will find a spurious association between Y and X. The non-mathematical explanation for this phenomenon is as follows: we know both X and Y can influence Z, say, positively; if we observe a positive change in Z, we know either X or Y is the possible cause, but we are uncertain of which it might be. However, if we then know that X has also changed, then the likelihood that Y has also changed is less than that Y has not changed, so a negative relation between X and Y would be observed. Mathematically speaking, X and Y are independent unconditionally, but they become dependent conditional on Z. In this scenario, Z acts as a collider because the two arrows (one from X and the other from Y) go toward it, so Z blocks the pathway from X to Y (and Y to X). However, statistical adjustment of Z will open this path, and X and Y will then become correlated.

3.2.3 Example of a Complex DAG

The simple scenario in Figure 3.4 does not do justice to the value of DAGs. Consider the DAG in Figure 3.6—suppose we want to estimate the true effect of X on Y. Which variables should be measured and adjusted for? As

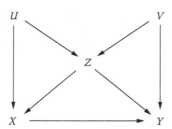

FIGURE 3.6
A complex example of DAG.

discussed before, variables to be adjusted for are confounders; that is, the adjustment of these variables can block the backdoor paths from X to Y. The most obvious confounder in Figure 3.5 is Z, as there is a backdoor path: $X \leftarrow Z \rightarrow Y$. Following the same principle, U and V are also confounders for the estimation of the causal effects of X on Y. The question is, do we need to adjust for all three variables? For instance, suppose that it would take a great effort and many resources to measure either U or V. The objective is to determine the minimum set of confounders needed for statistical adjustment. We then note that when Z is blocked (i.e., statistically adjusted for), the backdoor path from X to U, Z and Y is also blocked. As a result, blocking Z will block two backdoor paths from X to Y. The same applies to V. When Z is blocked, the backdoor path from X to Z, V and Y is also blocked. However, does this mean that the adjustment of Z would be sufficient to block *all* the backdoor paths? The answer is no because Z is also a collider for U and V. When Z is adjusted for, a new backdoor path from X to U, V and Y is opened, and therefore the minimum set of confounders is either Z and U or Z and V.

3.3 Direct and Indirect Effects

In the previous section we noted that DAGs are very useful for identifying confounders that need to be adjusted for in the statistical analysis. However, does this mean that non-confounding variables should not be adjusted for? For instance, in Figure 3.4b, Z is on the causal pathway from X to Y, so Z is not a confounder. Does this mean that Z must not be adjusted for? What would happen if Z is adjusted for? The adjustment of variables on the causal path is a contentious issue not only in epidemiology but also in other disciplines. One justification for this practice is the partition of direct and indirect effect, and this is very common in the SEM literature. The path from X to Y in Figure 3.4b is interpreted as the direct effect of X on Y, and the path from X to Z to Y is the indirect effect of X on Y. To estimate the former, we need to adjust for an intermediate variable between X and Y. This practice is also known as *mediation* analysis in the social sciences (MacKinnon 2008). We will return to this topic in Chapter 7 on the statistical adjustment in the foetal original hypothesis.

3.4 Summary

This chapter provides a concise introduction to path diagrams and DAGs, and these tools will be frequently used in later chapters. Discussion of path diagrams and the estimations of their parameters can be found in any SEM textbook. A more comprehensive discussion of DAGs and their application in epidemiology can be found in the chapters of two epidemiological textbooks (Glymour 2006; Glymour and Greenland 2008).

4

Mathematical Coupling and Regression
to the Mean in the Relation between
Change and Initial Value

4.1 Introduction

The relationship between initial disease status and subsequent change following treatment has attracted great interest in medical and dental epidemiology. It is an amazing example of how a deceptively simple question has managed to confuse generations of researchers.

In randomised controlled trials, the main research question is usually whether or not the observed change in disease status, assessed by observed change in overall means of the health outcome before and after treatment, can be attributed to the treatment. In clinical practice, when treatments are proven to be effective, differential baseline effects are also of interest to many clinicians because sometimes one might seek to identify subgroups of patients who may benefit more from one treatment than another. For instance, suppose that two drugs—A and B—show similar mean treatment effects for hypertension in blood pressure (*BP*) reduction but there is differential baseline effect in patients given drug A and not in those given drug B. Clinicians might decide to give drug A to patients who suffer the disease more seriously, especially if complications and/or costs of A and B differ.

Many clinical studies claim to show that patients with greater disease severity at baseline respond better to treatment. For instance, in medicine, the reduction in blood pressure amongst patients taking anti-hypertensive medication was found to correlate positively with baseline blood pressure (Gill et al. 1985). Weight loss following gastric surgery in obese patients was shown to correlate positively with the initial weight of the patients (Halverson and Koehler 1981). More examples can be found in the book by Björn Andersen (1990) on the methodological errors in medical research. In dentistry, numerous studies have claimed to show that baseline disease status is associated with the treatment outcome, and reviews of the problems with the statistical analyses in such studies can be found in previous publications (Tu et al. 2004a, 2004b, 2005a, 2006c).

In the statistical literature, the relation between baseline disease severity and treatment effect has a generic name, *the relation between change and initial value* (Blomqvist 1977), because treatment effect is evaluated by measuring the change of variables from their initial (baseline) values. In psychology, it is also well known as *the law of initial values* (Jin 1992). However, testing the relation between change and initial value using correlation or regression has long been criticised by many statisticians as problematic. Two methodological concerns known as *mathematical coupling* (Archie 1981; Moreno et al. 1986; Stratton et al. 1987; Andersen 1990; Tu et al. 2002) and *regression to the mean* have been raised as the causes of the problem in testing the relation between change and initial value (Oldham 1962; Altman 1982, 1991a, 1991b; Blomqvist 1987; Hayes 1988; Kirkwood and Sterne 2003).

Mathematical coupling occurs when one variable directly or indirectly contains the whole or part of another, and the two variables are then analysed using correlation or regression (Archie 1981). As a result, the statistical procedure of testing the null hypothesis—that the coefficient of correlation or the slope of regression is zero—might no longer be appropriate (Andersen 1990), and the results need to be interpreted cautiously (Archie 1981; Andersen 1990; Tu et al. 2002). Regression to the mean occurs with any variable that fluctuates within an individual or a *population* (the latter is sometimes overlooked, as we will point out later in this chapter) either due to measurement error and/or physiological variation (Bland and Altman 1994a, 1994b; Yudkin and Stratton 1996; Fitzmaurice 2000; Morton and Torgerson 2003). For instance, one is likely to obtain different readings of systolic *BP* for the same individual when a series of measurements are made over a short time period. This can be attributed to either the 'true' underlining *BP* fluctuating around a mean value (i.e., assuming *BP* can be taken without measurement error), or the device used to measure *BP* (or the person who uses the device) not being entirely reliable (this is treated as measurement error) or both.

Several alternative statistical methods have been proposed in the clinical and statistical literature to overcome problems in testing the relation between change and initial value using correlation or regression. In this chapter, we first provide a critical review of the proposed solutions to testing the relation between change and initial value in the statistical and psychological literature. Then a widespread conceptual confusion around regression to the mean within the statistical literature and a popular misconception about the *correct* analysis of the relationship between change and initial value in certain scenarios is clarified. It is then demonstrated how to derive a correct null hypothesis, and a new statistical method is proposed. In the final section we demonstrate that another common practice of categorising baseline values into groups and testing the differences in changes between these groups, whilst likely to avoid the problem of mathematical coupling, still suffers serious drawbacks and can yield misleading conclusions due to regression to the mean.

4.2 Historical Background

The problem of mathematical coupling among variables in correlation or regression analyses has long been noticed since these statistical techniques were first developed in the late nineteenth century (Pearson 1897; Yule 1910). Pearson (1897) first warned against the careless use of correlation with ratio variables when the two ratios shared a common denominator. Ever since, many statisticians have issued warnings regarding the interpretation of the relationship between mathematically coupled variables (Gumble 1926; Baker 1942; Simon 1954; Kronmal 1993). Pearson defined *spurious correlation* to be 'a correlation that is produced by a process of arithmetic, and not by any organic relationship between the quantities dealt with' (Aldrich 1995).

So, what is the spuriousness in spurious correlation? As Neyman (1952) argued, it is not that the correlation itself is spurious but that the interpretation can be spurious and misleading. In other words, when a positive correlation between change in pocket depth and baseline pocket depth is interpreted to mean that, on average, the greater the pre-treatment pocket depth the greater the treatment effect can be obtained, this interpretation is potentially spurious.

4.3 Why Should Change Not Be Regressed on Initial Value? A Review of the Problem

Although many authors warn against correlating or regressing change on initial value, it is far from clear what the problem is with this practice. The most commonly given reason is that testing the relation between change and initial value using correlation or regression suffers regression to the mean, but why does testing the relation between change and initial value using correlation or regression suffer regression to the mean? The most popular answer given in the literature is that regression to the mean is caused by biological variation and/or measurement error in the assessment of initial values. For example, Healy (1981) argued thus: suppose the true (unobserved) initial value is X and the true change is D; then the true follow-up value is $Y = X - D$. Assuming that the measurement errors e_X and e_Y are uncorrelated with X, Y and each other, the observed initial value is $x = X + e_X$, and the observed follow-up value $y = Y + e_Y$, with the observed change $d = x - y = D + e_X - e_Y$. Therefore, testing the relation between change and initial value is to test the relation between x and d.

Since e_X occurs in both x and d, their correlation is likely to be positive. If change is defined as $y - x$ (as in some psychological literature), the correlation between change and initial value will tend to be negative. As this error term occurs in both change and initial value, testing the relation between change and initial value using correlation or regression is biased. As a result, the problem of regression to the mean in testing the relation between change and initial value seems to be caused only by measurement error in the initial value and, consequently, the whole problem is reduced to the problem of measurement error in initial value. Therefore, any statistical method that aims to correct the bias caused by measurement error in the initial value might provide a solution.

4.4 Proposed Solutions in the Literature

4.4.1 Blomqvist's Formula

Blomqvist (1977) devised a formula to correct for measurement errors in initial values to obtain an unbiased estimate of regression slopes in analysing the relation between change and initial value. Blomqvist's formula is given as (Blomqvist 1987)

$$b_{\text{true}} = \frac{b_{\text{observed}} - k}{1 - k}, \tag{4.1}$$

where b_{true} is the true regression slope, b_{observed} is the observed regression slope, and k is the ratio of the measurement error variance for x (e_x^2) and the observed variance of x (s_x^2). If b_{true} is close to zero, it is then assumed that there is no evidence that change (e.g., reduction in BP) is dependent upon initial values (e.g., baseline BP). As one assumption behind ordinary least squares regression is that covariates are measured without errors, Blomqvist's formula corrects for the bias caused by measurement error and/or biological variation in the initial values. This formula requires an independent (external) estimate of the error variance, which is often obtained by measuring initial values repeatedly in a short interval before the intervention is administered.

4.4.2 Oldham's Method: Testing Change and Average

Oldham (1962) warned against testing the relation between treatment effect of anti-hypertensive therapy and patients' initial blood pressure. One of his arguments, which has been used repeatedly by others (Andersen 1990;

Altman 1991b), is that if we generate two series of independent random numbers x and y with the same standard deviation, a strong correlation ($1/\sqrt{2} \approx 0.71$) between $x - y$ and x is observed. Following previous notation, let x be the observed pre-treatment (initial) value and y the observed post-treatment value. The Pearson correlation between change ($x - y$) and pre-treatment value (x) is (Oldham 1962)

$$Corr(x - y, x) = r_{x-y,x} = \frac{s_x - r_{xy}s_y}{\sqrt{s_x^2 + s_y^2 - 2r_{xy}s_x s_y}}, \qquad (4.2)$$

where s_x^2 is the variance of x, s_y^2 is the variance of y, and r_{xy} is the correlation between x and y.

If s_x^2 and s_y^2 are equal, Equation 4.2 reduces to $r_{x-y,x} = \sqrt{(1 - r_{xy})/2}$. This formula shows that unless r_{xy} is unity, $r_{x-y,x}$ will never be 0. When r_{xy} is less than 1, the correlation between baseline and change, $r_{x-y,x}$, will always be positive. As r_{xy} is unlikely to be unity in practice, $r_{x-y,x}$ will never be 0. When r_{xy} is close to zero; that is, there is poor correlation between pre- and post-treatment values, the positive association between baseline and change will be large. Therefore, if both x and y are measured with large error, r_{xy} will be much less than 1, and we will find a large and positive $r_{x-y,x}$.

The solution proposed by Oldham (1962) did not deal with the problem of measurement error in initial values directly. Oldham suggested that testing the hypothesis that treatment effects are related to initial values should be carried out by testing the association between change and the average of the pre- and post-test values, and *not* with the initial values. For instance, if pre-treatment BP is denoted as x, and post-treatment BP as y, BP reduction after patients are given anti-hypertensive medication will be $x - y$, and the average BP will be $(x + y)/2$. To address whether or not greater baseline BP is related to greater BP reduction following treatment, Oldham's method tests the correlation between $x - y$ and $(x + y)/2$ instead of testing the correlation between $x - y$ and x. The Pearson correlation between change and average is (Oldham 1962)

$$Corr[x - y, (x + y)/2] = \frac{s_x^2 - s_y^2}{\sqrt{(s_x^2 + s_y^2)^2 - 4r_{xy}^2 s_x^2 s_y^2}}, \qquad (4.3)$$

where s_x^2 is the variance of x, s_y^2 is the variance of y, and r_{xy} is the correlation between x and y.

The numerator in Equation 4.3 indicates that Oldham's method is a test of the differences in the variances between two repeated measurements, where the two variances may be correlated. If there is no difference in the variances of pre-treatment BP (x) and post-treatment BP (y), the correlation using Oldham's method will be zero; that is, the treatment effect (BP reduction) does not depend upon baseline *BP*. The rationale behind Oldham's method is that if, on average, greater *BP* reduction can be obtained for greater baseline *BP*, the post-treatment *BP* values will become *closer* to each other; that is, the variance of post-treatment *BP* (s_y^2) will *shrink* and become smaller than that of pre-treatment *BP* (s_x^2). In other words, if there is a *differential* treatment effect (i.e., a greater or smaller treatment effect can be achieved in subjects with greater disease severity), the variance of post-treatment *BP* will be different from that of pre-treatment *BP*. As a result, if there is no difference in the two variances, there is no evidence for a *differential* treatment effect across the levels of baseline values. In other words, Oldham's method is to test the equivalence of two variances, and this test has been proposed as early as the 1930s by Morgan (1939) and Pitman (1939).

4.4.3 Geometrical Presentation of Oldham's Method

Using the basic geometric tools introduced in Chapter 2, we know that when x and y are two independent random variables (i.e., the correlation between x and y is expected to be zero), the angle between their vector representations x and y is $\pi/2$ radians (or 90°), and these two vectors are therefore orthogonal; that is, $x \perp y$. If x and y have the same variance, then vectors x and y have the same length (i.e., $\|x\| = \|y\|$), and the length of $x - y$ (i.e., the SD of $x + y$) will be $\sqrt{2}\|x\|$, and the angle between $x - y$ and x will be $\pi/4$ radians (Figure 4.1a). From elementary trigonometry, $cos(\pi/4) = 1/\sqrt{2} \approx 0.71$.

Applying vector geometry to Oldham's method, it becomes apparent that $x + y$ and $x - y$ are orthogonal vectors *if and only if* x and y have equal lengths. This property holds irrespective of the correlation between x and y (Figure 4.1b). Therefore, the angle between vectors $x + y$ and $x - y$ is determined by the length of x and the length of y; that is, the correlation between variables $x + y$ and $x - y$ is determined by the variances of x and y.

4.4.4 Variance Ratio Test

Following Oldham's (1902) arguments, testing the differential baseline effects seems to be testing the equivalence of the variances between pre- and post-treatment measurements. Based on the same assumptions, Geenen and Van der Vijver (1993) proposed the variance ratio s_x^2/s_y^2 as an appropriate test by assessing the equality of the correlated variances, yielding a statistic that follows the *t*-distribution with $n - 2$ degrees of freedom (Guilford and Fruchter 1973), which is non-significant if the variances are similar:

$$t = \frac{\left(s_x^2 - s_y^2\right)\sqrt{n-2}}{2s_x s_y \sqrt{1 - r_{xy}^2}},$$
(4.4)

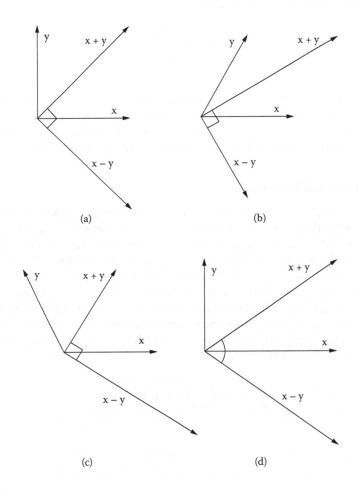

FIGURE 4.1

Vector geometry of Oldham's method. (a) When the correlation between two variables x and y is zero, their corresponding vectors, **x** and **y**, will be orthogonal; that is, the angle between the two vectors is π/2 radians. (b) When the correlation between x and y is positive, the angle between **x** and **y** will be less than π/2. (c) When the correlation between x and y is negative, the angle between **x** and **y** will be greater than π/2. (b and c) When the two vectors **x** and **y** have equal length, the angle between vectors **x** + **y** and **x** − **y** will always be π/2, irrespective of the angle between **x** and **y** (a). (d) When the two vectors x and y have unequal length, the angle between vectors **x** + **y** and **x** − **y** will no longer be π/2.

where s_x^2, s_y^2 and r_{xy} are as defined previously. Let $d = x - y$, $s = x + y$ and r_{ds} be the correlation between d and s; Equation 4.4 is exactly equivalent to the one proposed by Maloney and Rastogi (1970):

$$t = \frac{r_{ds}\sqrt{n-2}}{\sqrt{1-r_{ds}^2}} \qquad (4.5)$$

Like Oldham's method, this test assumes that the error variances in x and y are independent and equal, and the variances of x and y follow a normal distribution. This test has been used as a two-sided test to assess whether or not there is any baseline effect (Geenen and Van der Vijver 1993).

4.4.5 Structural Regression

Structural regression has been proposed in the psychological literature (Myrtek and Foerster 1986) to test the relation between the unobserved, true X and Y, by correcting for measurement error in the observed variables x and y. If the regression slope for Y regressed on X is less than 1 (i.e., the regression slope for $X - Y$ regressed on Y is greater than zero), it indicates that the change $(X - Y)$ is dependent upon baseline value (X). In biostatistics, structural regression is also used for the correction for measurement error (Dunn 2004). By assuming that the variances of measurement errors of X (e_X) and Y (e_Y) are equivalent, the maximum likelihood estimate of the regression slope for Y on X, $\hat{\beta}$, is (Dunn 2004)

$$\hat{\beta} = \frac{s_y^2 - s_x^2 + \sqrt{\left(s_y^2 - s_x^2\right)^2 + 4s_{xy}^2}}{2s_{xy}}, \qquad (4.6)$$

where s_{xy} is the covariance of x and y. Denoting $\mathbf{M}$ as the covariance matrix of x and y, the eigenvalues of $\mathbf{M}$, λ, are derived by solving $\mathbf{M} - \lambda\mathbf{I} = 0$ (where $\mathbf{I}$ is the identity matrix):

$$\lambda_1 = \frac{s_y^2 + s_x^2 + \sqrt{\left(s_y^2 + s_x^2\right)^2 - 4(s_x^2 s_y^2 - s_{xy}^2)}}{2}$$

and

$$\lambda_2 = \frac{s_y^2 + s_x^2 - \sqrt{\left(s_y^2 + s_x^2\right)^2 - 4(s_x^2 s_y^2 - s_{xy}^2)}}{2}.$$

In fact, $\hat{\beta}$ is the slope of the first principal component of x and y (Cleary 1986; Myrtek and Foerster 1986), and can be estimated by

$$\frac{\lambda_1 - s_x^2}{s_{xy}}$$

(Selvin 1994):

$$\frac{\lambda_1 - s_x^2}{s_{xy}} = \frac{\frac{s_y^2 + s_x^2 + \sqrt{\left(s_y^2 + s_x^2\right)^2 - 4(s_x^2 s_y^2 - s_{xy}^2)}}{2} - s_x^2}{s_{xy}} = \frac{s_y^2 - s_x^2 + \sqrt{\left(s_y^2 - s_x^2\right)^2 + 4s_{xy}^2}}{2s_{xy}}$$

From a geometrical perspective, as long as the correlation between x and y (r_{xy}) is not zero (therefore s_{xy} is not zero), the slope of the first principal component will be unity *if and only if* the variances of x and y are equivalent. Thus, using structural regression to test the slope of the first principal component ($\hat{\beta}$) is again to test the equivalence of the variances of x and y.

4.4.6 Multilevel Modelling

Another approach is to use multilevel modelling (Goldstein 1995; Blance et al. 2005). Multilevel modelling estimates individual trajectories for each subject by treating the initial and post-treatment values as the lower level and subjects as the upper level. A covariate *Time* (i.e., the initial and follow-up occasions) is used to model the changes over the observation period. The estimated intercepts and slopes for *Time* within those individual trajectories are assumed to follow a multivariate normal distribution, and the correlation between the variance of the intercept and the variance of the slope in the multilevel model indicates the relation between baseline disease status (intercept) and changes (slope). The variances of the intercept and slope are also known as *random effects*, and multilevel models are sometimes known as *random effects models*. Using *BP* as an example, the two-level model is written as

$$(BP)_{ij} = \beta_{0ij} + \beta_{1j}Time_{ij} + e_{ij} \tag{4.7}$$

Multilevel modelling can estimate the variances of β_0 and β_1, namely, u_0^2 and u_1^2, respectively, and the covariance between β_0 and β_1, namely, u_{01}. The correlation between change and initial value is therefore $u_{01}/(u_0 * u_1)$.

When *Time* has only two occasions (i.e., pre- and post-treatment), some constraints need to be imposed to estimate u_{01} due to the lack of sufficient degrees of freedom (Blance et al. 2005). It is noted that four random effects (or random variables) are actually estimated in Equation 4.7: u_0^2, u_1^2, u_{01} and e_{ij}. However, with two blood pressure measurements (pre- and post-treatment), there are only three degrees of freedom (two observed variances and one observed covariance of the two *BP* measurements); that is, at most we can only estimate three random effects in Equation 4.7. As a result, either u_0 or e_{ij} needs to be constrained to zero, and for the sake of interpretation, the latter is constrained to zero. There is no need for this constraint when there are more than two repeated *BP* measurements.

It should also be noted that different codings of *Time* will yield different results (Blance et al. 2005). For instance, when *Time* is coded as 0 (baseline) and 1 (follow-up), testing the correlation between intercept and slope is equivalent to testing $r_{x-y,x}$ because the intercept variance is the variance of *x*, and the slope variance is the variance of $x - y$; when *Time* is centred, such as -0.5 (baseline) and 0.5 (follow-up), testing the correlation between intercept and slope is equivalent to Oldham's method because the intercept variance is the variance of $(x + y)/2$, and the slope variance is the variance of $x - y$; when *Time* is coded as -1 (initial) and 0 (post-treatment), testing the correlation between intercept and slope is equivalent to testing $r_{x-y,y}$ because the intercept variance is the variance of *y*, and the slope variance is the variance of $x - y$.

An advantage of multilevel modelling over other approaches is that this method can be applied to more than two measurement occasions, and other covariates can be entertained into the models. A good introduction to multilevel modelling for epidemiologists can be found in Hox (2002) and Twisk (2006).

4.4.7 Latent Growth Curve Modelling

Another approach similar to multilevel modelling is latent growth curve modelling (LGCM) within the framework of structural equation modelling (Bollen and Curran 2006; Duncan et al. 2006; Tu et al. 2008a; Tu et al. 2009a), and the analysis is undertaken using structural equation modelling software packages such as Amos, Lisrel, EQS and Mplus. From a statistical viewpoint, LGCM is equivalent to multilevel models for longitudinal data analysis, and therefore it can also be used for testing the relation between changes and initial values. Book-length discussions of LGCM can be found in Bollen and Curran (2006) and Duncan et al. (2006).

In Section 4.4.6, the variances of the intercept and slope for *Time* in multilevel models of longitudinal data are treated as random effects, but in LGCM they are explicitly treated as latent variables. For instance, the two *BP* measurements can be expressed as two simultaneous equations:

$$BP_0 = 1 * intercept + 0 * slope + e_0 \qquad (4.8)$$

$$BP_1 = 1 * intercept + 1 * slope + e_1 \qquad (4.9)$$

where BP_0 is the initial blood pressure and BP_1 the post-treatment *BP*. The residual errors e_0 and e_1 are e_{ij} in Equation 4.7. LGCM can estimate the variances and covariance for *intercept* and *slope*, but with the same consideration for the number of degrees of freedom in Section 4.4.6; that is, e_0 and e_1 have to be constrained to zero. It should also be noted that different parameterizations for the regression coefficients for *slope* will yield different covariance estimates between *intercept* and *slope*, just as different codings for *Time* in Equation 4.7 yields different results. For example, if Equations 4.8 and 4.9 are written as

$$BP_0 = 1 * intercept + (-0.5) * slope + e_0 \qquad (4.10)$$

$$BP_1 = 1 * intercept + (0.5) * slope + e_1, \qquad (4.11)$$

it is noted that $BP_1 - BP_0 = slope$, and $\frac{1}{2}(BP_1 + BP_0) = intercept$. As a result, Equations 4.10 and 4.11 yield the same results as Oldham's method. A less technical introduction to LGCM can be found in our previous publication (Tu et al. 2009a).

4.5 Comparison between Oldham's Method and Blomqvist's Formula

It has been claimed that Oldham's method is biased toward a negative association if (1) the individuals have been selected on the basis of high initial values, or (2) the 'true' treatment effect differs across individuals (Hayes 1988; Kirkwood and Sterne 2003). Therefore, it has been claimed that Blomqvist's formula performs better than Oldham's method for these two circumstances. However, whilst it is correct that Oldham's method will indeed lead to biased results in scenario 1, we have shown in our previous study that the argument surrounding scenario 2 is a misunderstanding (Tu and Gilthorpe 2007). In fact, Oldham's method gives rise to correct results for scenario (2), whereas Blomqvist's formula does not. In our previous study, we undertook simulations to clarify this misunderstanding (Tu and Gilthorpe 2007).

Results from our simulations demonstrated that in scenario (1), a subgroup with greater baseline values than the whole sample was selected, and the variance of the subgroup post-treatment values will be greater than that of the subgroup baseline values; Oldham's (1962) method therefore shows a spurious inverse association between treatment effect and baseline. In contrast, Blomqvist's formula in general yields unbiased results and therefore performs better than Oldham's method.

However, in scenario (2), whilst Blomqvist's formula showed a zero regression slope, it has been argued that when true treatment effects differ across subjects, Oldham's method would give rise to a misleading negative association when the true treatment effect is *not* associated with true baseline values (Hayes 1988; Kirkwood and Sterne 2003). The expected zero correlation or regression coefficient between the unobserved true baseline values X and true treatment effects D is *misinterpreted* as evidence to show that there is no *differential* treatment effect across the levels of baseline values. As Oldham pointed out in his reply to critics (Garside 1963; Oldham 1963), the relationship between $D = X - Y$ and X is potentially deceiving and should be interpreted cautiously. The zero correlation between D and X does not mean that treatment effects were not related to severity of baseline diseases. On the contrary, there is a reverse baseline effect (i.e., for greater baseline values, lesser treatment effects will be achieved) because the variance of y is greater that that of x. The correct interpretation of the zero correlation between D and X is that the response of the patients to treatment was so *heterogeneous* that the correlation between D and X becomes zero, and this is why the correlation between D and X is close to zero. In other words, the zero regression slope simply means that it is not possible to predict the amount of changes in, say, blood pressure, for individual patients using their baseline blood pressure. However, it is the difference in variances between the post-treatment value Y and the baseline value X that is crucial to the interpretation of the relationship between treatment effects and baseline values, not the correlation or regression slope between treatment effect and baseline. As early as 1933, the distinguished statistician and economist Harold Hotelling, and later his student the influential economist Milton Friedman, had issued warnings about the potential misinterpretation of the relation between changes and initial values (Hotelling 1933; Friedman 1992).

Another way to reveal that the expected zero regression slope given by Blomqvist's formula in scenario 2 should not be interpreted as evidence of no differential baseline effect on the treatment is to regress changes on true follow-up values Y. Since changes are not related to baseline values, there is no reason that changes should then be related to follow-up values. Our simulations showed that whilst Blomqvist's formula showed zero regression slope for D regressed on X, it nevertheless showed a negative slope for D regressed on Y.

4.6 Oldham's Method and Blomqvist's Formula Answer Two Different Questions

The misinterpretation of different results between Oldham's (1962) method and Blomqvist's formula in scenario 2 is due to overlooking the full impact of regression to the mean in testing the relation between change and initial value. As discussed in previous sections, some authors mistakenly reduce the problem to testing the relation between changes and initial values to the problem of measurement error (e_X) in the true initial value X and consider it the only cause of regression to the mean. Therefore, any method to correct for the bias caused by e_X is believed to be a sufficient solution. Blomqvist's formula provides an unbiased estimate for the regression slope (i.e., the expected changes in *BP* per 1 unit increase in baseline *BP*) because it adjusts for the bias in regression slope caused by measurement errors in baseline *BP* (or any covariate). As one assumption for ordinary least squares regression is that covariates are measured without errors, Blomqvist's formula gives the correct estimate of regression slope by accommodating covariate (baseline) errors. However, another cause of regression to the mean is the heterogeneous response to treatment, which does *not* bias the estimate of regression slope (but causes misleading interpretation of the regression slope), and therefore this will not be corrected by Blomqvist's formula. Blomqvist's formula does not answer the question of whether or not there is a differential baseline effect, which is addressed by Oldham's method (and other approaches as discussed in Section 4.4).

To help clarify this crucial distinction, it is useful to briefly revisit how Sir Francis Galton first discovered regression to the mean more than one century ago (Galton 1886).

4.7 What Is Galton's Regression to the Mean?

Influenced by his famous cousin Charles Darwin, Galton was interested in the heritance of human intelligence. However, owing to the lack of a precise measure of intelligence, he turned to measurable traits such as body heights (Galton 1886; Stigler 1997). He invited families to submit their body height to his laboratory. As males on average are taller than females, all female heights were multiplied by 1.08, and then he plotted the average of both parents' heights against their offspring's heights (Senn 2003; Hanley 2004). He found that, although adult children of tall parents were still taller than most people, they were generally shorter than their parents; that is, they were closer to the mean height of the population. On the other hand, adult children of short parents, whilst still short, were on average taller than their parents; that is, they were closer to the mean height of the population. Galton named this phenomenon *regression toward mediocrity*, and we know it today as regression to the mean.

It is important to note that regression to the mean in Galton's study was not the relation between repeated measurements of heights on the *same* individuals (where regression to the mean might occur, though it is generally quite small) but the relation between measurements of body heights *across genera-tions* (i.e., between parents and their adult children). Consequently, in Galton's study, regression to the mean was not only caused by measurement errors of individuals' heights but also by the underlying genetic and environmental factors related to the growth of body height. Suppose that all parents' and their adult children's heights were measured twice, one week apart. This would provide information about the magnitude of measurement error and/ or biological fluctuation in height (though the latter is probably ignorable), and this information could, for example, be used in Blomqvist's formula for the adjustment of measurement errors in the height of both parents and their adult children. However, this would not eliminate regression to the mean in the analysis of the relation between body heights across generations. Compared to the variation in body heights occurring *across generations*, due to biological and/or environmental factors, the variation in measurement errors would be small and have modest impact on the correlation between heights of parents and their adult children.

The phenomenon of regression to the mean has been much discussed in medical research. For instance, in the hierarchy of evidence-based medicine, results from randomised controlled trials (RCTs) are considered a higher level of evidence than observational studies because control groups in RCTs pro-vide estimates for the treatment effects caused by regression to the mean and other potential bias such as placebo and Hawthorne effects. When patients with higher values of blood pressure are recruited into an intervention trial, their average blood pressure might decline at the re-assessment, even whilst the intervention has no genuine effect on reducing *BP*. It should be noted that, in this example, the reduction in blood pressure in the control group is caused by both measurement errors in baseline *BP* and measurement errors in the physiological fluctuation in *BP*. An instrument with greater reliability and precision for *BP* measurement can certainly reduce the effect of regres-sion to the mean caused by measurement errors but cannot eliminate the effect caused by physiological fluctuation; that is, even if blood pressure were measured with an instrument without error, it still varies hour by hour and day by day. In later chapters we will come across more examples of how regression to the mean can give rise to misleading interpretation of statisti-cal analysis.

4.8 Testing the Correct Null Hypothesis

In a book on methodological errors in medical research, Andersen (1990) has argued that, due to mathematical coupling, the null hypothesis for testing the correlation between $x - y$ and x ($r_{x-y,x}$) is no longer zero. However, he did

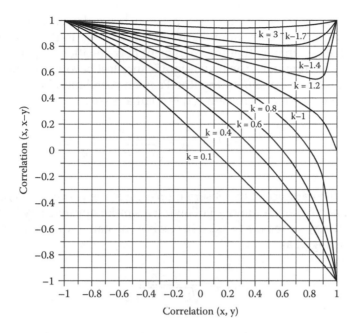

FIGURE 4.2
The possible range of the correlation between x and $x - y$ is related to the correlation between x and y. For example, when the correlation between x and y is 0.2, the possible range for the correlation between x and x – y is about –0.1 to 1. (Modified from Figure 1 in Tu, Y.K., Baelum, V., Gilthorpe, M.S., *European Journal of Oral Sciences*, 113, p. 281, 2005. With permission.)

not explain how to derive a correct null hypothesis. In a short note, Bartko and Pettigrew (1968) showed that the range of $r_{x-y,x}$ is restricted by the correlation between x and y (r_{xy}), and the range of $r_{x-y,x}$ is generally not between –1 and 1 (Figure 4.2). Therefore, the usual null hypothesis that the correlation coefficient is zero is no longer appropriate to test the relation between change and initial value, and the associated P-values given by statistical packages are misleading. In our previous study, we showed how to derive the appropriate null hypothesis and then to compare the observed correlation between change and initial value against the correct null hypothesis and proposed a new approach to testing the appropriate null hypothesis (Tu et al. 2005a).

4.8.1 The Distribution of the Correlation Coefficient between Change and Initial Value

The proposed approach is based on studying the distribution and plausible range of the correlation coefficient between changes and baseline values. Suppose the baseline value is denoted as x and the post-treatment value as *y*, then change is $x - y$. As discussed previously (Andersen 1990), the problem with testing the correlation between x and $x - y$ is that the standard null hypothesis—that is, that the coefficient of correlation ($r_{x,x-y}$) is zero—is erroneous, and, therefore, the usual significance test becomes inappropriate. Previously, it has been shown that the Pearson correlation between change $(x - y)$ and the pre-treatment value (x) is (Oldham 1962)

$$Corr\left[x, x-y\right] = r_{x,x-y} = \frac{s_x - r_{xy}s_y}{\sqrt{s_x^2 + s_y^2 - 2r_{xy}s_xs_y}}, \tag{4.2}$$

where s_x^2 is the variance of the observations x, s_y^2 is the variance of y, and r_{xy} is the correlation between x and y. Following a similar approach by Bartko and Pettigrew (1968), suppose $s_x = ks_y$, where k is a constant (>0), and Equation 4.2 can be rearranged as

$$r_{x,x-y} = \frac{k - r_{xy}}{\sqrt{k^2 + 1 - 2kr_{xy}}}, \tag{4.12}$$

which shows that the values of $r_{x,x-y}$ are affected by k and r_{xy}. As we know that $\infty > k > 0$ and $1 \geq r_{xy} \geq -1$, we can plot $r_{x,x-y}$ against k and r_{xy} (Figure 4.3). When $r_{xy} = -1$, $r_{x,x-y}$ will always be 1. When r_{xy} increases, the range of $r_{x,x-y}$ becomes greater. When $r_{xy} = 0$, the range of $r_{x,x-y}$ is between 0 ($k \to 0$) and 1 ($k \to \infty$). When r_{xy} is 1, there is a singularity and only three scenarios exist: for $k = 1$, $r_{x,x-y}$ is *undefined*; for any $k < 1$, $r_{x,x-y} = -1$; and for any $k > 1$, $r_{x,x-y} = 1$.

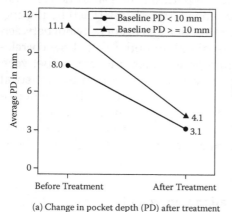
(a) Change in pocket depth (PD) after treatment

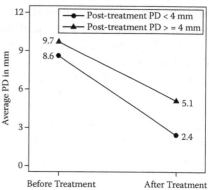
(b) Change in pocket depth (PD) after treatment

FIGURE 4.3
(a) The changes in probing depth (PD) after treatment in the two groups divided according to their baseline PD; (b) the changes in PD after treatment in the two groups divided according to their PD reduction.

From Figure 4.3, it is obvious that the plausible range of $r_{x,x-y}$ is not between 1 and –1, as we would expect for a *normal* correlation coefficient. Moreover, when $r_{xy} < 0$, then $r_{x,x-y}$ will be always greater than zero. This illustrates that the usual null hypothesis; that is, that the correlation coefficient is zero, is no longer appropriate due to $r_{x,x-y}$ being constrained by k and r_{xy}; consequently. the associated *P*-values are misleading.

4.8.2 Null Hypothesis for the Baseline Effect on Treatment

The correct null hypothesis for the baseline effects on treatment must take into consideration k and r_{xy}. As many statisticians such as Hotelling (1933) and Oldham (1962) argued previously, if changes in variables are related to their baseline values, there will be changes in the variances of the variables. For instance, if changes in systolic blood pressure (*SBP*) are indeed related to baseline *SBP*; that is, the more hypertensive subjects on average obtain greater *SBP* reduction when treated, the variance of post-treatment *SBP* will become smaller than that of baseline *SBP*. Therefore, for a given r_{xy}, the correct null hypothesis for the test of $r_{x,x-y}$ is the value of $r_{x,x-y}$ when k is unity. It follows from Equation 4.12 that when $k = 1$, the expected value of $r_{x,x-y}$; that is, the null hypothesis for the test of baseline effects on treatment is

$$H_0 = \sqrt{\frac{1-r_{xy}}{2}} . \tag{4.13}$$

For instance, when $r_{xy} = -0.3$, the null hypothesis for $r_{x,x-y}$ is 0.806; when $r_{xy} = 0$, the null hypothesis for $r_{x,x-y}$ is 0.71; or when $r_{xy} = 0.7$, the null hypothesis for $r_{x,x-y}$ is 0.387. Therefore, to test $r_{x,x-y}$, we need to know r_{xy} and take this into consideration.

4.8.3 Fisher's Z-Transformation

Pearson's correlation coefficients are not normally distributed (Cohen and Cohen 1983; Dawson and Trapp 2001), and it was Ronald Fisher who used his great geometric insight to obtain the distribution of the correlation coefficient (Fisher 1915). To compare any two correlation coefficients, we need to use Fisher's z-transformation:

$$z_r = \frac{1}{2} \ln\left(\frac{1+r}{1-r}\right). \tag{4.14}$$

This transformation follows a normal distribution with standard error = $1/\sqrt{n-3}$, and the following expression for the z-test can be used (Cohen and Cohen 1983; Dawson and Trapp 2001):

$$z = \frac{z_r(r) - z_r(\rho)}{\sqrt{1/(n-3)}}, \tag{4.15}$$

where r is the correlation coefficient of the sample, and ρ is the correlation coefficient to be tested against. The null hypothesis that $r - \rho = 0$ is evaluated by testing $z_r(r) - z_r(\rho) = 0$. To compare the sample correlation $r_{x,x-y}$ with the correct null value correlation derived, we first use Equation 4.14 to transform the two correlation coefficients and then carry out the significance testing using Equation 4.15.

4.8.4 A Numerical Example

Data kindly made available by Dr. Lars Laurell are used to demonstrate how to use this approach to test for baseline effects on treatment (Falk et al. 1997). In a group of 203 infrabony lesions treated with guided tissue regeneration, the correlation between baseline probing pocket depth (PPD) and PPD reduction, $r_{x,x-y}$, was found to be 0.648. Incorrect significance testing (i.e., where the null hypothesis correlation is assumed to be zero) shows this value to be highly significant ($P < 0.0001$). However, as the correlation between baseline and post-treatment clinical attachment level (CAL) values, r_{xy}, was 0.343, the correct value for the null hypothesis test, as derived by Equation 4.9, is 0.573, not zero. Application of Fisher's z-test shows that

$$z = \frac{z_r(0.648) - z_r(0.573)}{\sqrt{1/(203-3)}} = \frac{0.772 - 0.652}{\sqrt{1/200}} = 1.68.$$

Referring the value $z = 1.68$ to the standard normal distribution yields, for a two-sided test, $P = 0.09$, which is not significant at the 5% level.

4.8.5 Comparison with Alternative Methods

To evaluate the performance of our proposed test, we undertook a study (see Tu et al. 2005a for details) by searching original data on the treatment effect of guided tissue regeneration and enamel matrix protein derivatives in infrabony defects (see the glossary in Chapter 1 for explanations of these surgical procedures). In summary, four major periodontal journals (*Journal of Periodontology, Journal of Clinical Periodontology, Journal of Periodontal Research,* and *International Journal of Periodontics and Restorative Dentistry*) were searched for all human studies that had appeared between 1986 and 2003, which fulfilled the criteria that they either contained actual measurements of PPD or CAL for each treated defect or allowed these measurements to be derived from other clinical parameters. All data extracted from the identified publications were re-analysed to test for baseline effects on treatment using (a) the conventional approach; that is, to test the correlation between the change and baseline value against the incorrect null hypothesis that the correlation coefficient is zero; (b) Oldham's (1962) method; that is, to test the correlation between change $(x - y)$ and the average $(x+y)/2$; (c) the new approach proposed in this book using Fisher's z-transformation; that is, to test the correlation between change and baseline values against the null hypothesis derived by Equation 4.9; and (d) computer simulations to provide information regarding the robustness of our proposed approach in the circumstances of a moderate sample size since the sample size in most periodontal studies is often small.

Our study (Tu et al. 2005a) showed that the conventional approach (i.e., testing the correlation between changes and initial values) suggested significant correlation between treatment effects, such as PPD reduction and CAL gain, and baseline PPD and CAL in most published studies. However, Oldham's (1962) method, the proposed new approach and simulation all showed this correlation to be significant in only a few studies. Testing the correct null hypothesis yielded comparable results to Oldham's method and simulations (Tu et al. 2005a). This approach has been used in research on alcohol addiction, and its results are again comparable to Oldham's method (Gmel et al. 2008). A recent study on *BP* changes following exercise also used this approach to correct for regression to the mean and found the previous evidence on the relation between changes in *BP* and baseline values to be spurious (Taylor et al. 2010).

4.9 Evaluation of the Categorisation Approach

Another commonly used approach to test the relation between change and baseline value (especially in dental epidemiology) is to categorise outcomes into subgroups according to threshold values, such as the mean or median outcome value, or otherwise predetermined values. For example, PPD and/or CAL are categorised according to predefined values such as 4 mm or 6 mm (Pihlstrom et al. 1981; Lindhe et al. 1984; Kaldahl et al. 1988; Loos et al. 1989; Zitzmann et al. 2003; Harris 2004), and researchers subsequently compare treatment effects in terms of changes in PPD/CAL across the two (or across more) such subgroups (Pihlstrom et al. 1981; Lindhe et al. 1984; Kaldahl et al. 1988; Loos et al. 1989). A related subgroup comparison approach is to categorise the outcomes into subgroups according to their response to treatment, followed by a comparison across these subgroups of baseline values (Heden et al. 1999; Pontoriero et al. 1999). These two approaches will be henceforth called the *categorisation approach*.

Even though the approach of categorising lesions according to their initial disease status or their response to treatment does not use either correlation or regression to analyse the data, thereby avoiding the effects of mathematical coupling, this approach is still questionable due to the effects of regression on the mean. The effects are best illustrated using an example in which data were made available by Dr. Laurell, pertaining to the treatment of 203 infrabony defects using guided tissue registration (GTR; Falk et al. 1997).

Defects were divided into two groups according to their baseline pocket depth value (mean = 9.03 mm, SD = 1.86 mm) such that group one consisted of defects with baseline PPD < 10 mm, and group two comprises defects with baseline PPD > 10 mm. The mean baseline PPD of defects in each group was 8.0 mm and 11.1 mm, respectively, and the mean post-treatment PPD was 3.1 mm and 4.1 mm, respectively. It follows that the mean pocket reduction was 4.9 mm and 7.0 mm, respectively. This indicates that deeper pockets had better treatment responses. This is shown in Figure 3.4a, which demonstrates that differences in the mean PPD between groups became smaller following GTR treatment.

However, when the same defects were divided according to their post-treatment values, the results became quite different. The post-treatment PPD had a mean of 3.4 mm with SD of 1.63 mm. Defects with post-treatment PPD < 4 mm formed group one, and those with baseline PPD > 4 mm formed group two. The mean post-treatment PPD of defects in each group was 2.4 mm and 5.1 mm, respectively, and the mean baseline PPD was 8.6 mm and 9.7 mm, respectively. The mean pocket reduction was thus 6.2 mm and 4.6 mm, respectively. This indicates that shallower pockets had much better treatment responses than did deeper pockets. This is illustrated in Figure 3.4b, which shows that differences in the mean PPD between groups was greater after GTR treatment, indicating that the deeper the baseline PPD, the less pocket reduction achieved.

Contradictory conclusions were therefore reached from the same data, depending on how the defects were categorised. Regression to the mean is the source of this contradiction. It should be noted that the reanalysis of these data in Section 4.8.4 indicated that there was no association between the baseline PPD values and the treatment response.

We conducted computer simulations to evaluate to what extent and under which circumstances the categorisation approach can, due to regression to the mean, cause spurious results regarding the relationship between baseline disease severity and treatment effects. It was shown that the smaller the correlation between baseline and follow-up values, the greater the impact of regression to the mean; that is, the greater the spurious association observed. Also, as sample sizes increase, the spurious association became more likely to be statistically significant.

4.10 Testing the Relation between Changes and Initial Values When There Are More than Two Occasions

Oldham's (1962) method and testing the correct null hypothesis approach can only use the first and final measurements when repeated measurements are made on more than two occasions. In such scenarios, multilevel modelling and latent growth curve modelling, as discussed in Sections 4.4.6 and 4.4.7, respectively, seem to offer better approaches as they can utilise the intermediate measurements to estimate the correlation between overall change and initial value. These methods can also use intermediate measurements to estimate potential measurement errors in the repeated measurements, giving rise to a more accurate estimation. We use a data set of 20 boys with four radiographic measurements of their ramus length (ramus is the vertical component of the lower jaw and its growth is related to lower facial height) at ages 8, 8.5, 9 and 9.5 years (Elston and Grizzle 1962) for illustration. The research question is whether growth in the ramus between ages 8 and 9.5 is related to the ramus length at age 8; that is, whether boys with greater length of ramus at age 8 will go on to have greater or less growth in ramus length. Figure 4.4 shows the growth trajectories of the 20 boys. To utilise all four ramus measurements rather than the first and final ones, we used the statistical software package MLwiN to carry out a multilevel analysis, and the results are shown in Figure 4.5.

The variable *length* is the repeated measures of ramus length, *id* is the identifier for each boy, and *age* are the chronological ages subtracted by the baseline

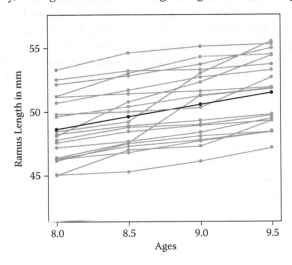

FIGURE 4.4
Growth trajectories for ramus between ages 8 and 9.5 in a group of 20 boys.

$$\text{length}_{ij} \sim N(XB, \Omega)$$

$$\text{length}_{ij} = \beta_{0ij}\text{cons} + \beta_{1j}\text{age}_{ij}$$

$$\beta_{0ij} = 48.666(0.573) + u_{0j} + e_{0ij}$$

$$\beta_{1j} = 1.896(0.263) + u_{1j}$$

$$\begin{bmatrix} u_{0j} \\ u_{1j} \end{bmatrix} \sim N(0, \Omega_u) : \Omega_u = \begin{bmatrix} 6.424(2.070) \\ -0.654(0.696)\ 1.232(0.440) \end{bmatrix}$$

$$\begin{bmatrix} e_{0ij} \end{bmatrix} \sim N(0, \Omega_e) : \Omega_e = \begin{bmatrix} 0.194(0.043) \end{bmatrix}$$

$-2^*loglikelihood(IGLS\ Deviance) = 234.533(80$ of 80 cases in use)

FIGURE 4.5
Results from multilevel analysis using statistical software MLwiN.

age of 8 years (i.e., *age* = 0, 0.5, 1, 1.5). Results in the fixed effects section showed that, on average, ramus grew 1.9 mm per year, and the average ramus length was 48.67 mm. The random effects for the intercept and slope were 6.424 and 1.232, respectively, and their covariance was −0.654; that is, their correlation was $-0.654/\sqrt{(6.424 * 1.232)} = -0.232$, indicating that boys with greater ramus length at age 8 had smaller increases in ramus length between ages 8 and 9.5. The confidence intervals can be obtained using the Markov chain Monte Carlo (MCMC) estimation procedure in MLwiN, and the 95% credible intervals from 100,000 simulations were between −2.757 and 0.752.

As discussed in Section 4.4.6, however, to obtain a correct relation between changes and initial values, we need to reparametrise *age* by subtracting its mean; that is, by subtracting 0.75 from *age*, yielding the new variable *cage* = (−0.75, −0.25, 0.25, 0.75). Results from multilevel analysis using *cage* are shown in Figure 4.6. The fixed effects section showed that, on average, ramus grew 1.9 mm per year, and the average ramus length at the age of *8.75* years was 50.09 mm. The random effects for the intercept and slope were 6.135 and 1.232, respectively, and their covariance was 0.269; that is, their correlation was $-0.269/\sqrt{(6.135 * 1.232)} = 0.098$, indicating that boys with greater ramus length at age 8 seemed to have very slightly greater increases in ramus length between ages 8 and 9.5, although this relation was not statistically significant. The same analysis can also be carried out using latent growth curve modelling.

4.11 Discussion

The misunderstanding of differences between Blomqvist's and Oldham's (1962) approaches impacts not just the testing of the relation between change

$$\text{length}_{ij} \sim N(XB, \Omega)$$

$$\text{length}_{ij} = \beta_{0ij}\text{cons} + \beta_{1j}\text{cage}_{ij}$$

$$\beta_{0ij} = 50.087(0.556) + u_{0j} + e_{0ij}$$

$$\beta_{1j} = 1.896(0.263) + u_{1j}$$

$$\begin{bmatrix} u_{0j} \\ u_{1j} \end{bmatrix} \sim N(0, \Omega_u): \Omega_u = \begin{bmatrix} 6.135(1.951) \\ 0.269(0.657)\ 1.232(0.440) \end{bmatrix}$$

$$\begin{bmatrix} e_{0ij} \end{bmatrix} \sim N(0, \Omega_e): \Omega_e = \begin{bmatrix} 0.194(0.043) \end{bmatrix}$$

$-2*loglikelihood(IGLS\ Deviance) = 234.532(80\ \text{of}\ 80\ \text{cases in use})$

FIGURE 4.6
Results from multilevel analysis using statistical software MLwiN.

and initial value. For instance, there was a debate regarding how to investigate the underlying risk as a source of heterogeneity in meta-analyses (Brand 1994; Senn 1994; Sharp et al. 1996; Thompson et al. 1997; Van Houwelingen and Senn 1999). The approach of Oldham's method has again been criticised for yielding misleading results when there is variation in the treatment effects across different clinical trials (Sharp et al. 1996; Thompson et al. 1997). However, this criticism is based on the same arguments used by Hayes (1988) and others to criticise Oldham's method in testing the relation between change and initial value in scenario 2, and it has been shown in this chapter that this criticism is not tenable. If a treatment really works better in patients with greater underlying risk of developing a disease, the variance of the log odds in the treatment groups will be smaller than the variance of the log odds in the placebo groups. If these two variances remain similar, the treatment effects are not related to the underlying risk in the placebo groups. However, the problem with meta-analyses is more complex (Van Houwelingen and Senn 1999) since sample sizes and protocols are usually different across different trials.

Another conceptual confusion is around the distinction between mathematical coupling and regression to the mean (Myles and Gin 2000). Mathematical coupling is more often encountered in clinical research. For instance, within anaesthesiology and critical care on oxygen supply and oxygen delivery, both indices are derived using complex formulae with some common components (see page 89 in Myles and Gin (2000) for the equation). When the shared components in both indices are measured with error, testing their interrelationship using correlation or regression yields biased results, just as measurement errors in baseline values causes biased estimates in the testing of a relation between change and initial value. However, when both are measured without error, mathematical coupling still prevails. Whilst approaches to correct for measurement errors can give rise to an unbiased estimate of regression slopes (Moreno et al. 1986; Stratton et al. 1987), for coupled variables, such methods cannot estimate the *strength* of the relation (i.e., whether or not a relation is statistically significant) because the null hypothesis might no longer be zero. This more general situation is analogous to using Blomqvist's formula to correct for the bias in the relation between change and initial value. Correcting for measurement errors in mathematically coupled variables might yield unbiased predictions of oxygen consumption for a given level of oxygen delivery, but it remains uncertain whether or not the relation between oxygen consumption and delivery is statistically significant; that is, whether the increased oxygen delivery will physiologically increase oxygen consumption.

One limitation in the application of both Oldham's (1962) method and the proposed new strategy is that these methods are only valid if measurement error variances of the baseline and post-treatment values differ negligibly. This assumption might not always be true in periodontal research. For instance, the measurement errors of PPD might be associated with the true (unobserved) PPD. Thus, when the mean PPD is reduced following treatment, the measurement error variance for post-treatment PPD might be smaller than that for pre-treatment PPD. Consequently, even with no genuine change in the variance of the *true* PPD between measurement occasions, there is a difference in the variances of the *observed* PPD. Another limitation is that the new approach and Oldham's method are only suitable for study designs with two measurements.

Problems related to the categorisation approach have been occasionally discussed in the statistical literature (Hotelling 1933; Friedman 1992; Stigler 1999). Nevertheless, many researchers are not aware of those problems, and misleading conclusions are drawn from results using the categorisation approach. For instance, in December 2007, a report on the association between children's cognitive performance and their parents' socioeconomic status (SES) drew the national media's attention. The authors had categorised the children according to both their cognitive test results at the age of 3 years and their parents' SES, and found that those children with good test results and poor SES performed less well at the subsequent tests at the age of 5 years. In contrast, those children with poor test results and good SES at the age of 3 years performed better at the age of 5 years. As a result, it was concluded that parents' SES has an important impact on children's cognitive development at such early ages. Although the conclusions may be correct, the statistical analysis nevertheless suffers regression to the mean as demonstrated in this chapter. We have commented on this example elsewhere (Tu and Law 2010).

5

Analysis of Change in Pre-/Post-Test Studies

5.1 Introduction

Analysis of change from baseline is probably the most popular study design in medical and epidemiological research. If the study subjects are randomly allocated to different treatment groups, such as in randomised controlled trials, the comparisons of changes amongst groups are relatively straight-forward; a few statistical issues are occasionally discussed, around which methods give rise to unbiased estimates, and some discussions focus on which statistical methods yield the greater statistical power. In contrast, if the subjects come from naturally assigned groups, such as those in observational studies, then making comparisons of changes from the baseline usually requires making some crucial assumptions that are quite often hard to ascertain; this warrants considerably more discussion around the statistical process and the interpretation of results.

5.2 Analysis of Change in Randomised Controlled Trials

Randomised controlled trials (RCTs) are widely recommended as the most useful study design to generate reliable evidence. There are textbooks and journal articles devoted to the subject of assessing RCTs, and a consensus statement (CONSORT) has been published and updated regularly by an international team to give guidance on the design, conduct and publication of RCTs (Moher et al. 2001). However, a recent article examined the quality of RCTs in dental research according to several criteria, and the results were discouraging (Montenegro et al. 2002), revealing that the quality of these RCTs frequently failed to reach recommended standards.

An important issue frequently overlooked in evaluations of the quality of RCTs in dental research is sample size and hence, study power. The power of a hypothesis test relates to the probability of rejecting the null hypothesis when the alternative hypothesis is true (Dawson and Trapp, 2001). When a test incorrectly fails to reject the null hypothesis, it is known as Type II error. Power is defined as $(1 - \beta)$, where β is the probability of Type II error (Moye 2000). The lack of power has been addressed previously (Hujoel and DeRouen 1992; Gunsolley et al. 1998), although it is still not common practice for published trials to declare clearly how they determine power and sample size before the start of each trial. Moreover, it is relatively unknown to clinical researchers that the statistical analyses used to compare differences in treatment effects can have substantial impact on study power.

In the statistical and epidemiological literature, it has been shown that the analysis of covariance (ANCOVA) has a greater statistical power and gives a more precise estimation of treatment effects than testing change scores or percentage scores in RCTs with two measurements (i.e., pre- and post-intervention). Consequently, ANCOVA has been recommended as the preferred method for analyses of data from RCTs (Senn 1997, 2006; Vickers 2001; Twisk and Proper 2004). However, a major concern about using ANCOVA arises from the imbalance of baseline values across different treatment groups, and this might give rise to a biased estimate of treatment difference between groups due to regression to the mean (RTM; Cohen and Cohen 1983; Campbell and Kenny 1999; Boshuizen 2005; Forbes and Carlin 2005). In theory, properly implemented randomisation will ensure that all initial characteristics (such as gender, age, smoking status and baseline disease severity) are approximately equal across groups, though in reality there might be some differences in these characteristics between groups simply due to random sampling errors.

Suppose the efficacy of a new drug for reduction of blood pressure (*BP*) is tested in an RCT and, after randomisation, patients in the treatment group are found to have a higher initial systolic blood pressure (*SBP*) than those in the placebo group. The issue is that, due to RTM, it is very likely that patients in both groups might show *SBP* reduction even though the new drug (and the placebo) has no genuine treatment effect. This is because those participating are usually recruited due to their (initially) higher than normal *SBP*. Either due to measurement error and/or physiological fluctuation of *SBP*, the average *SBP* of these patients taken on the second occasion might be reduced even without any intervention given between the two measurements. If the treatment group has an overall *higher* mean *SBP* than the placebo group, the phenomenon of RTM might become more prominent and, therefore, patients in the treatment group might show a greater change in blood pressure from baseline than those in the placebo group, whilst both the drug and the placebo have no genuine effect.

The proponents of ANCOVA, however, argue that if there is an imbalance in the baseline values due to random sampling errors in the randomisation process, the adjustment of baseline values in ANCOVA will actually remove the bias caused by RTM and give rise to correct findings (Senn 1997, 2006; Vickers and Altman 2001); that is, that the new drug is no better than the placebo. In contrast, using change scores will give a wrong impression that the new drug works. Critics of the use of ANCOVA in such instances argue that if the imbalance in baseline blood pressure between the treatment and placebo groups cannot be attributed to chance (which is always unknown), the adjustment of baseline values using ANCOVA will be an overadjustment and, in contrast, testing change scores will give a correct result (Cohen and Cohen 1983; Campbell and Kenny 1999; Mohr 2000; Boshuizen 2005).

In this chapter we examine carefully the role of ANCOVA in both randomised and non-randomised (i.e., observational) studies, considering statistical power and the potential for bias.

5.3 Comparison of Six Methods

In a previous study, we conducted simulations to determine (1) whether there were substantial differences in the statistical power amongst various statistical methods for the analysis of change, (2) how pre- and post-treatment correlation affects the performance of each method, and (3) whether or not treatment effects are associated with baseline disease severity (Tu et al. 2005b). The hypothetical research question is to detect whether a new but expensive treatment achieves better treatment outcomes than a conventional one. We choose the comparison between guided tissue regeneration (GTR) and conventional flap operation in the treatment of periodontal infrabony defects for our illustration and simulations, as there have been numerous studies in the previous literature to compare GTR to conventional treatments since the concept of GTR was introduced, though many may severely suffer from inadequate statistical power.

The hypothetical study design is to randomly allocate the patients to treatment (GTR) and control groups, and each patient contributes only one lesion. The treatment outcome is clinical attachment level (CAL) gain, though this could also be probing pocket depth (PPD) reduction. The pre-treatment CAL (CAL_0) is 9 mm with standard deviation (SD) of 2 mm, based on original data available from the literature related to GTR (Cortellini and Tonetti 2000) and enamel matrix protein derivatives (Esposito et al. 2009). Three SDs of post-treatment CAL (CAL_1) are considered: 2 mm, 1.5 mm and 1 mm. If there is no difference in the SD between *precal* and *postcal*, the treatment effects are not dependent on the baseline disease levels (see Chapter 4). The treatment effect is 4 mm for the treatment group and 2 mm for the control group; that is, (a) there is 2 mm difference in the performance of the two treatments. Six commonly used univariate or multivariate statistical methods of analysing change are used to test whether this 2 mm difference can be efficiently detected.

5.3.1 Univariate Methods

5.3.1.1 Test the Post-Treatment Scores Only

It has been proposed that if the intra-individual variation and/or measurement error is large in RCTs, using post-treatment scores only can improve precision and study power (Blomqvist and Dahlén 1985) because the baseline values are supposed to be balanced (due to randomisation). That is, one can use the *t*-test for the trial with two groups only, or analysis of variance (ANOVA) for trials with more than two groups, to test differences in means of post-treatment values between the treatment and control groups. The rationale behind this method is that the commonly used change scores (see the next method) contain greater measurement errors. Suppose the variance of true but unobserved CAL_0 is δ_0^2 and the variance of its measurement errors is σ_0^2, and the variance of true CAL_1 is δ_1^2 and the variance of its measurement errors is σ_1^2. The variance of the change in CAL becomes $(\rho_{12}\delta_0\delta_1 + \sigma_0^2 + \sigma_1^2)$, where ρ_{12} is the true correlation between CAL_0 and CAL_1. As the variance contains two measurement error terms, some consider it less reliable than the post-treatment values (Blomqvist and Dahlén 1985). In the simulations, a two-sample *t*-test is used to compare the means of post-treatment values of the outcome variable CAL in the two groups.

5.3.1.2 Test the Change Scores

This is probably the most commonly used method in clinical research. The change scores are derived by subtracting post-treatment values from the pre-treatment values; that is, *attachment level gain* = pre-treatment clinical attachment level (CAL_0) – post-treatment clinical attachment level (CAL_1). The *t*-test is used to test the differences in the means of change score between treatment and control groups. It is worth noting that testing the interaction between treatment *group* and measurement *occasion* using repeated measures ANOVA will achieve exactly the same results as testing change scores using the *t*-test (Huck and McLean 1975).

5.3.1.3 Test the Percentage Change Scores

The percentage change scores are derived by dividing the change score by the pre-treatment value: *percentage attachment level gain* = (*attachment level gain*/CAL_0) * 100. The *t*-test is then used to test the difference in the means of percentage change scores between the treatment and control groups.

5.3.1.4 Analysis of Covariance

Commonly, multiple regression analysis is used to analyse the differences in post-treatment values with the adjustment of pre-treatment values. This is given the special name of ANCOVA, though it is not always called this explicitly within the clinical literature. The following regression model is employed:

$$CAL_1 = b_0 + b_1 CAL_0 + b_2 group + e, \tag{5.1}$$

where *group* is a categorical variable for the control (coded 0, the reference) and treatment groups (coded 1), and *e* is the residual errors. Attention is given to b_2, which, if significant, is deemed to show that there is genuine difference in the treatment outcome between treatment and control groups. It should be noted that it is similarly possible to determine the effect of *group* in a related regression model (Laird 1983):

$$(CAL_0 - CAL_1) = \beta_0 + \beta_1 CAL_0 + \beta_2 group + e, \tag{5.2}$$

where the dependent variable is replaced by the *change score*. Although regression Equation 5.2 is more widely used in clinical research, most researchers are not aware that these two models are related, with $\beta_1 = 1 - b_1$, $\beta_2 = -b_2$ and the *P*-value for b_2 or β_2 being the same (Laird 1983).

5.3.2 Multivariate Statistical Methods

The four univariate statistical methods can only use one variable such as post-treatment CAL or use a summary of two variables such as change in CAL and percentage change in CAL as their outcome variable. In contrast, multivariate methods treat more than one variable as outcomes, which is why they are *multivariate* methods.

5.3.2.1 Random Effects Model

This approach is also known as a mixed effects model, multilevel model, or hierarchical linear model. The model used in this study is

$$CAL_{ij} = b_0 + b_1 occasion_{ij} + b_{2j} group_j + b_3 occasion_{ij} * group_j, \tag{5.3}$$

where CAL_{ij} is CAL measured on occasion *i* for subject *j*, b_{0ij} is the mean baseline CAL for treatment group, *occasion* is the time when CAL is measured, *group* is a categorical variable for the control (coded 0, the reference) and treatment groups (coded 1), and *occasion * group* is an interaction term derived by multiplying *occasion* by *group*. Attention is given to b_3, which, if significant, is deemed to show that there is genuine difference in the treatment outcome between treatment and control groups. This is the simplest two-level random effects models of repeated measures (Gilthorpe et al. 2000, 2001; Hox 2002). There are two ways to model the random effects in Equation 5.3:

1. A random intercept model: Each patient is allowed to have his or her own intercepts (i.e. baseline values) estimated, and therefore $b_0 = \beta_0 + u_{0j} + e_{0ij}$, where b_0 is the grand mean for the baseline value in the control group, u_{0j} is the random effects (i.e., variations) for intercepts, and e_{0ij} is the residual errors.

2. A random slope model: Each patient is allowed to have his or her own intercepts and treatment effects estimated; that is, $b_0 = \beta_0 + u_{0j} + e_{0ij}$ and $b_1 = \beta_1 + u_{1j}$. Usually, the covariance between u_0 and u_1 is also estimated. However, this is not possible for the model in Equation 5.3, because there are only two measurements for each patient. Recall that in Chapter 4, Section 4.4.6 on the multilevel modelling approach to testing the relationship between changes and baseline values, due to the limited number of degrees of freedom, it is not possible to estimate all the random effects, and we encounter the same problem here. One solution is that we constrain e_{0ij} to be zero, as we did in Section 4.4.6, and in this case the random effects approach is equivalent to testing change scores. Therefore, in our simulation study, we used the random intercept model instead.

5.3.2.2 Multivariate Analysis of Variance

MANOVA (multivariate analysis of variance) was the most popular multivariate method before random effects modelling and before powerful desktop computers became available (Bray and Maxwell 1985; Ekstrom et al. 1990). This approach has been used and discussed extensively by psychologists in analyses of repeated experimental measures and longitudinal studies. MANOVA treats pre- and post-treatment CAL simultaneously as outcomes and *group* as a covariate; that is, an explanatory variable. The null hypothesis is

$$H_0 = \begin{pmatrix} \mu_{x1} \\ \mu_{y1} \end{pmatrix} = \begin{pmatrix} \mu_{x0} \\ \mu_{y0} \end{pmatrix},$$

where μ_{x1} is the mean of pre-treatment values in the treatment group, μ_{y1}, is the mean of post-treatment values in the treatment group, μ_{x0}, the mean of pre-treatment values in the control group, and μ_{x0}, the mean of post-treatment values in the control group. In the pre-/post-test design with two groups, the multivariate test statistic for MANOVA, Hotelling's T^2, is given as (Stevens 2002)

$$T^2 = \frac{n_0 n_1}{n_0 + n_1} \left(\mu_{x1} - \mu_{x0}, \mu_{y1} - \mu_{y0} \right) \mathbf{S}^{-1} \begin{pmatrix} \mu_{x1} - \mu_{x0} \\ \mu_{y1} - \mu_{y0} \end{pmatrix}, \tag{5.4}$$

where n_0 is the sample size of the control group, n_1 is the sample size of the treatment group, and the matrix $\mathbf{S}$ is given as

$$S = \frac{W_0 + W_1}{n_0 + n_1 - 2},$$

where

$$W_0 = \begin{bmatrix} ss_{x0} & ss_{xy.0} \\ ss_{yx.0} & ss_{y0} \end{bmatrix}, \text{ and } W_1 = \begin{bmatrix} ss_{x1} & ss_{xy.1} \\ ss_{yx.1} & ss_{y1} \end{bmatrix}.$$

The sum of squares, ss_{x0}, for the control group (coded as 0) is defined as

$$\sum_{j=1}^{n_0} \left(X_{0j} - \overline{X}_0 \right)^2,$$

where X_{0j} are the pre-treatment values and $\overline{X}_0$ is the group mean of the pre-treatment values in the control group. The sum of squares, ss_{y0}, for the control group is defined as

$$\sum_{j=1}^{n_0} \left(Y_{0j} - \overline{Y}_0 \right)^2,$$

where Y_{0j} are the post-treatment values and $\overline{Y}_0$ is the group mean of the post-treatment values in the control group. The sum of the cross-product, $ss_{xy.0} = ss_{yx.0}$, for the control group is defined as

$$\sum_{j=1}^{n_0} \left(X_{0j} - \overline{X}_0 \right) \left(Y_{0j} - \overline{Y}_0 \right).$$

The sum of squares, ss_{x1}, for the treatment group (coded as 1) is defined as

$$\sum_{j=1}^{n_1} \left(X_{1j} - \overline{X}_1 \right)^2,$$

where X_{1j} are the pre-treatment values and $\overline{X}_1$ is the group mean of the pre-treatment values in the treatment group. The sum of squares, ss_{y1}, for the treatment group is defined as

$$\sum_{j=1}^{n_1} \left(Y_{1j} - \overline{Y}_1 \right)^2,$$

where Y_{1j} are the post-treatment values and $\overline{Y}_1$ is the group mean of the post-treatment values in the treatment group. The sum of the cross-product, $ss_{xy.1} = ss_{yx.1}$, for the treatment group is defined as

$$\sum_{j=1}^{n_1}\left(X_{1j}-\overline{X}_1\right)\left(Y_{1j}-\overline{Y}_1\right).$$

In studies with balanced design; that is, both treatment and control groups are assumed to have the same sample size $n_0 = n_1 = m$, where the total sample size $= n$, the means of pre-treatment values of the treatment and control groups are assumed to be equal; that is, $\mu_{x1} - \mu_{x0} = 0$. By defining $\mu_{y1} - \mu_{y0} = \delta$,

$$\mathbf{S} = \frac{1}{n-2}\begin{bmatrix} ss_{x0}+ss_{x1} & ss_{xy.0}+ss_{xy.1} \\ ss_{xy.0}+ss_{xy.1} & ss_{y0}+ss_{y1} \end{bmatrix} = \frac{n-1}{n-2}\begin{bmatrix} s_x^2 & s_{xy} \\ s_{xy} & s_y^2 - \dfrac{n\delta^2}{4(n-1)} \end{bmatrix},$$

where s_x^2 is the variance of the pre-treatment values, s_y^2, the variance of the post-treatment values, and s_{xy}, the covariance between the pre- and post-treatment values. As a result, Equation 5.4 can be shown to be

$$T^2 = \frac{n}{4}\begin{bmatrix} 0 & \delta \end{bmatrix}\left(\frac{n-2}{n-1}\right)\begin{bmatrix} s_x^2 & s_{xy} \\ s_{xy} & s_y^2 - \dfrac{n\delta^2}{4(n-1)} \end{bmatrix}^{-1}\begin{bmatrix} 0 \\ \delta \end{bmatrix}$$

$$= \frac{n}{4}\begin{bmatrix} 0 & \delta \end{bmatrix}\left(\frac{n-2}{n-1}\right)\left(\frac{1}{s_x^2(s_y^2-\dfrac{n\delta^2}{4(n-1)})-s_{xy}^2}\right)\begin{bmatrix} s_y^2 - \dfrac{n\delta^2}{4(n-1)} & -s_{xy} \\ -s_{xy} & s_x^2 \end{bmatrix}\begin{bmatrix} 0 \\ \delta \end{bmatrix}$$

$$= \frac{n}{4}\left(\frac{n-2}{n-1}\right)\left(\frac{1}{s_x^2(s_y^2-\dfrac{n\delta^2}{4(n-1)})-s_{xy}^2}\right)\begin{bmatrix} -\delta s_{xy} & \delta s_x^2 \end{bmatrix}\begin{bmatrix} 0 \\ \delta \end{bmatrix}$$

$$= \frac{n}{4}\left(\frac{n-2}{n-1}\right)\left(\frac{4(n-1)}{s_x^2(4(n-1)s_y^2-n\delta^2)-4(n-1)r_{xy}^2s_x^2s_y^2}\right)\delta^2 s_x^2$$

$$= \frac{n(n-2)\delta^2}{4(n-1)(1-r_{xy}^2)s_y^2-n\delta^2}$$

where r_{xy} is the correlation between pre-test and post-test values.

The F transformation of T^2 with p, $n - p - 1$ degrees of freedom is then (Stevens 2002)

$$F_{(p,n-p-1)} = \frac{n-p-1}{(n-2)p}T^2, \tag{5.5}$$

where p is 2 because there are two dependent variables. Therefore, F has 2 $(n - 3)$ degrees of freedom. Then, Equation 5.5 can be shown to be

$$F = \left(\frac{n-3}{(n-2)2}\right)\left(\frac{n(n-2)\delta^2}{4(n-1)(1-r_{xy}^2)s_1^2 - n\delta^2}\right) = \frac{1}{2}\left(\frac{n(n-3)\delta^2}{4(n-1)(1-r_{xy}^2)s_y^2 - n\delta^2}\right). \tag{5.6}$$

From Equation 5.6, it is clear that the statistical power of MANOVA is related to the treatment effect (δ), the variance of the post-treatment values (s_y^2) and the correlation between the pre- and post-treatment values (r_{xy}). The greater the treatment effect and/or the correlation between the pre-test and post-test values, the greater the statistical power. On the other hand, the smaller the variance of the post-test values, the greater the statistical power. Recall the discussion in Chapter 1 that the F-value is the square of the t-value, and the t-value for testing the regression coefficient b_2 for *group* in Equation 5.1 can be shown to have a mathematical relation with the F-value of MANOVA in Equation 5.6 (Tu 2005):

$$F_{(1,n-3)}\,(\text{ANCOVA}) = 2 * F_{(2,n-3)}\,(\text{MANOVA}).$$

From the tables of critical values for F (Stevens 2002), the F-value with 1, $n - 3$ degrees of freedom will always have a smaller P-value than $(1/2)*F$-value with 2, $n - 3$ degrees of freedom. Consequently, ANCOVA will always have greater power than MANOVA, irrespective of sample size.

5.5.3 Simulation Results

Results from our simulations showed a general pattern that conforms to theoretical expectations (Senn 1997). The power using post-treatment values only is unaffected by the correlation between the pre-treatment and post-treatment values ($r_{pre.post}$). The power of the other five statistical methods is dependent on $r_{pre.post}$, and as $r_{pre.post}$ increases, the power can exhibit a dramatic improvement. When $r_{pre.post}$ reaches 0.5, using change scores, percentage change scores, random effects modelling (REM) and MANOVA have comparable power to using the post-treatment values only. One interesting finding is that, typically, change scores and REM achieve comparable power throughout different $r_{pre.post}$ and sample sizes, and percentage change scores are slightly more powerful than change scores. Generally, the most powerful test is ANCOVA, which is well established and hence often stated in standard textbooks (Senn 1997; Bonate 2000; Vickers 2001; Vickers and Altman 2001). However, when $r_{pre.post}$ is small, the power of ANCOVA is slightly poorer than using the post-treatment values only, though higher than using the other methods. Whilst also known amongst some researchers, this is often overlooked, and formal statements are too easily made that ANCOVA is *always* the most powerful. Nevertheless, when $r_{pre.post}$ is moderate to large (negative or positive), ANCOVA is again the most powerful test. MANOVA has greater power than change scores, percentage change scores, and REM when $r_{pre.post}$ is low. In contrast, when $r_{pre.post}$ is high, MANOVA has less power than other methods.

For simulations of 10 patients per group; that is, a total study size of 20, although ANCOVA is the most powerful test for moderate-to-large $r_{pre.post}$, its power only ever reaches 80% for very large $r_{pre.post}$. For low correlations (0.1), using the post-treatment values yields the greatest power, though the power is only slightly above 50%. Using change scores or percentage change scores in general gives rise to unsatisfactory power to detect differences in the treatment effect between groups.

As the sample size increases to 20 in each group, the power of the six methods improves greatly. Only using the post-treatment values and ANCOVA give rise to acceptable power of over 80% for all values of $r_{pre.post}$. Using change scores, percentage change scores and REM yields 80% power when $r_{pre.post}$ is 0.5, and using MANOVA attains this level of power when $r_{pre.post}$ is only 0.3. When each group contains 30 patients, the six statistical methods always yield high power (>80%) to detect differences in the treatment effect between groups.

5.6 Analysis of Change in Non-Experimental Studies: Lord's Paradox

A similar but more complex problem with analysis of change occurs in non-experimental studies; that is, where subjects are not randomly allocated to different groups, which covers most epidemiological studies. For instance, in an observational study on the efficacy of water fluoridation in dental caries rates reduction, the risks of developing dental caries in children living in areas with water fluoridation were compared to those from areas without water fluoridation. Since living in areas with or without water fluoridation was not randomly allocated, if there is a difference in baseline dental caries rates between the two groups, it is uncertain whether or not this difference is due to random sampling errors or due to confounding factors such as socio-economic background.

The dilemma of whether or not baseline values should be adjusted for in non-randomised studies is extensively discussed within the social sciences. Inappropriate adjustment, which may lead to incorrect conclusions, is known within this field as Lord's paradox (Lord 1967, 1969), though it is less well known and hence, less well understood within epidemiology. A numerical example is used to illustrate the phenomenon of Lord's paradox.

Suppose a university authority wants to establish whether the food provided by its refectory has any effect on the weight of new students. In a prospective one-year observational study, 100 female and 100 male first-year students are randomly selected to participate. The students' weights are measured at the time of their entry to university and then again one year later. Results show that there was no substantial overall change in the weights of these students (on average), though some students gained weight whilst others lost weight. In subgroup analyses for male and female students separately, there was also no substantial overall change in weights between the two measurement occasions for each group (Table 5.1). The data were then subjected to statistical analyses by two statisticians.

The first statistician observed that there was no significant change in the mean values of weights between the two measurements for either female or male students using the paired t-test (Table 5.1) and no significant difference in weight change between female and male students using the two-sample t-test. He therefore concluded that the food provided by the refectory had no effect on the students' weight. In particular, there was no evidence of any differential effect by sex since neither group showed any systematic change. However, the second statistician decided that, because there was a significant difference in the initial weights (denoted $weight_1$) between female and male students, ANCOVA should be used to control for baseline differences. Therefore, the weight measured one year after entry into the university

TABLE 5.1

Hypothetical Data of 100 Female and Male Students' Weights Measured at the Time of Entry into the University and One Year Later

		Number	Minimum	Maximum	Mean	SD
Females	$weight_1$	100	33.4	79.4	53.7	7.5
	$weight_2$	100	32.0	80.5	53.3	9.0
Males	$weight_1$	100	55.9	90.8	71.3	8.4
	$weight_2$	100	54.1	90.6	71.9	9.1

Note: There was no significant difference between $weight_1$ and $weight_2$ in female or male students using paired t-test. $Weight_1$ = the initial weight measured at the time of entry into the university. $Weight_2$ = the weight measured one year later.

TABLE 5.2

Regression Analysis of Hypothetical Data
Using ANCOVA

Independent Variables	Coefficients	P-values
Intercept	7.152	0.014
Weight$_1$	0.861	0.001
Gender	3.425	0.007

Note: Dependent variable: weight$_2$.

(denoted weight$_2$) was utilized as the dependent variable in a regression model, with weight$_1$ and sex as independent variables. The model is thus

$$\text{weight}_2 = b_0 + b_1\text{weight}_1 + b_2\text{sex} + \varepsilon, \qquad (5.7)$$

where b_0 is the intercept, b_1 is the regression coefficient for weight$_1$, b_2 is the regression coefficient for the binary variable sex (female coded as 0 and male coded as 1) and ε is the random error term. In these analyses, weight$_1$ and sex are significant in the regression analysis (Table 5.2), and the second statistician therefore concluded that the food provided by the refectory affected the weights of the first-year students in the university, with male students gaining substantially more weight than female students.

The findings of the two statisticians are contradictory. This dilemma in the interpretation of the association between weight and sex is called Lord's paradox because it was Frederic M. Lord who brought attention to this issue in the social sciences (Lord 1967). The scenario of weight and sex was the original example in Lord's article, though the hypothetical data used here for illustration were our creation. In fact, as early as 1910, the same paradox was heatedly debated between the great statistician Karl Pearson and the famous welfare economist Arthur C. Pigou regarding the impact of parental alcoholism on the performance of children (see Chapter 1 in Stigler 1999).

Over the last few decades, Lord's paradox has been the subject of controversy in the statistical literature (Hand 1994), and the discussion around how to resolve this paradox can be found in the literature of the behavioural sciences and psychology (Cohen and Cohen 1983; Wainer 1991; Mohr 2000; Reichardt 2000). However, epidemiologists have only noticed this phenomenon very recently (Glymour et al. 2005).

5.6.1 Controversy around Lord's Paradox

5.6.1.1 Imprecise Statement of Null Hypothesis

One of the comments for the controversy in the Lord's paradox is that the null hypothesis is not explicitly formulated (Hand 1994). The null hypothesis being tested behind the *t*-test used by the first statistician in our hypothetical example is an *unconditional* statement that there is no change in weights between the two measurement occasions for either females or males. The hypothesis to be tested behind the ANCOVA is a *conditional* statement that if we select subgroups of females and males with *identical initial weights*, there is no difference in weights between females and males one year later. Some authors (Hand 1994; Campbell and Kenny 1999) argue that the confusion in Lord's paradox could be resolved were the null hypothesis always formulated explicitly *a priori*. If the null hypothesis to be tested is that there is no difference in the change of weights between female and male students with identical initial weights, the results given by ANCOVA are reasonable (Hand 1994).

However, if this *solution* satisfies statisticians, it is questionable that it will convince clinical researchers. The food in the refectory either caused differential weight changes between females and males or it did not, and the distinction between testing differences in weight changes between female and males *in general* (i.e., unconditionally) or between females and males *with identical weights* (i.e., conditionally) is not very helpful, or may even be confusing. One obvious question is, what does it mean by female and male students with identical initial weights? Suppose we only select students with body weight of 80 kg. It might not be difficult to recruit enough male students into our study, but we will have difficulty in finding females students with the same weight. On the other hand, if we select students with body weight of 55 kg, we will encounter the opposite dilemma.

Moreover, testing differences in the change of weights between female and male students with identical initial weights is probably considered pointless by clinical researchers because male students are *on average* heavier than females, and researchers usually want to know the average effects in the study population.

5.6.1.2 Causal Inference in Non-Experimental Study Design

In the hypothetical example of Lord's paradox, testing change scores using the *t*-test seemed to be a more reasonable approach than ANCOVA because the variable in question, sex, was *fixed*; that is, the sex of students could not be manipulated; the university students could not be randomly assigned to either female or male. However, in most non-experimental studies, although the participants are not randomly allocated to different groups, they are not fixed groups such as sex. Take the relation between dental caries and water fluoridation as an example. Suppose we find that children living in areas with water fluoridation have a lower initial caries rate and additionally are from more affluent families than children living in areas without water fluoridation. Also suppose there is evidence to show that socioeconomic background is related to children's oral health. Should the initial dental caries rate or the background socioeconomic circumstances be adjusted for? It is possible to take action to change both variables.

Many observational studies follow their subjects longitudinally to see whether there is any detectable difference in the outcomes between subgroups with different baseline characteristics. This is often done because either randomisation cannot be administered (for example, due to ethical reasons), or it is too difficult to administer. Consequently, statistical 'adjustments' are needed to accommodate potential differences in confounders between subgroups. However, to determine whether or not a variable is a genuine confounder is not always straightforward.

5.6.2 Variable Geometry of Lord's Paradox

The discussions on Lord's paradox, or, in general, the difference in results between ANCOVA and change scores, are mainly philosophical because both methods are well established and statistically valid. The difficulties arise due to study design rather than questionable statistical methodology. To illustrate the difference in the statistical outcome between ANCOVA and change scores, variable space geometry has been most often used (Lord 1967; Mohr 2000; Forbes and Carline 2005).

Following the example of weight gain and gender discussed in the previous section, the diagonal straight line in Figure 5.1, $y = x$, indicates a perfect correlation between weight$_1$ (x) and weight$_2$ (y); that is, there is no change

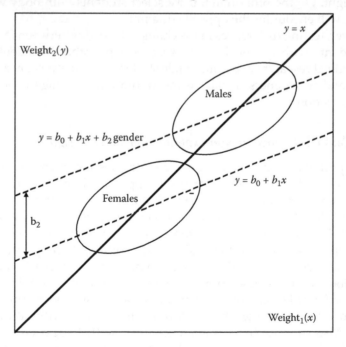

FIGURE 5.1
Geometrical illustration of Lord's paradox in variable space. The parallel dashed lines are the fitted regression lines for female and male students using ANCOVA.

in body weight for each student (female and male). Our hypothetical data will fall around this diagonal. Due to errors in the measurements and/or biological fluctuation in weights, the data will not form a perfect straight line but instead form two elliptical *clouds*. The spread of these *clouds* depends on the size of measurement errors and/or biological fluctuations. In other words, the correlation between x and y (and hence the regression slope for regressing y on x) is no longer unity. Using ANCOVA to fit the data allows the two groups to have two parallel regression slopes (the two dashed lines) though with different intercepts. As shown previously, the regression model for ANCOVA is

$$\text{weight}_2 = b_0 + b_1\text{weight}_1 + b_2\text{gender} + \varepsilon. \tag{5.7}$$

Testing the difference in the intercepts between females and males is equivalent to testing the regression coefficient for gender (b_2). It is obvious that the difference in the intercepts between females and males will be zero when either (1) these two groups are completely overlapped; that is, they have identical average initial and follow-up weights (and similar measurement error); or (2) b_1 is forced to be unity. In fact, testing the change scores is exactly equivalent to forcing b_1 to be unity.

5.6.3 Illustration of the Difference between ANCOVA and Change Scores in RCTs Using Variable Space Geometry

In RCTs, treatment and control group are supposed to have the same baseline characteristics such as baseline *SBP*. Although ANCOVA might have greater statistical power than testing change scores, both methods will obtain the same estimation of treatment differences (Figure 5.2). This is because any fitted regression lines for the treatment or control group have to pass through the group means, and in RCTs, the line connecting the two group means are parallel to the vertical axis. Therefore, the slopes (i.e., b_1) become irrelevant to the estimation of the difference in the two intercepts between the two groups (i.e., b_2). Testing post-treatment scores only can be seen as constraining b_1 to be zero, so the three univariate methods actually obtain the same estimation of treatment differences.

5.7 ANCOVA and *t*-Test for Change Scores Have Different Assumptions

For RCTs, ANCOVA is in general the preferred method for the analysis of change because it has greater statistical power. When the baseline values are balanced; that is, there is no group difference in the means of baseline values, ANCOVA and change scores should yield the same estimate of differences in

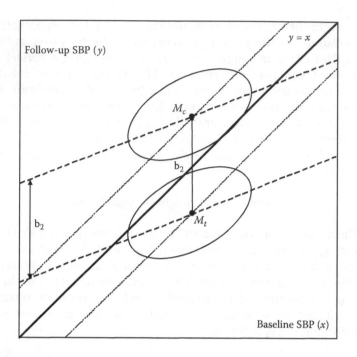

FIGURE 5.2
Geometrical illustration of ANCOVA and change scores in RCTs using variable-space geometry. The two parallel dashed lines are the fitted regression slopes for treatment and control groups using ANCOVA, and the two parallel dotted lines (which are forced to be unity) are the regression slopes for testing change scores using the t-test. The line connecting M_t (the group mean of treatment group) and M_c (the group mean of control group) is parallel to the vertical axis because these two groups have the same baseline blood pressure. Therefore, the vertical difference between the two parallel regression slopes (dashed lines) in ANCOVA is equal to that between the two regression slopes in testing change scores.

treatment effects. In real RCTs, baseline values may be slightly imbalanced due to random sampling variations, so the two tests may give rise to different estimates, though the difference is generally negligible. In observational studies, baseline values are usually not balanced, and the two tests may show contradictory results as demonstrated by Lord's paradox. In this section, we shall use directed acyclic graphs (DAG) to illustrate that there are different assumptions behind these two tests, and it is important to take these assumptions into account in the interpretation of results from ANCOVA or the t-test. In some statistical software packages for structural equation modelling, such as Amos, EQS, and Lisrel, it is possible to draw a path diagram on the computer screen to specify the causal relations amongst variables in the models, so they are also useful tools to illustrate the subtle differences in the assumptions between the two tests. Our previous study provides numerical examples for illustrating the differences in the assumptions and results between the t-test and ANCOVA (Tu et al. 2008a).

5.7.1 Scenario One: Analysis of Change for Randomised Controlled Trials

Suppose a hypothetical randomised controlled trial is conduced to test the efficacy of a new medication in the treatment of high blood pressure. Patients are randomly allocated to the treatment or the placebo control group. One of the outcome variables is the reduction in *SBP*, measured at baseline and one month later. A simple *t*-test in a regression analysis framework is given as

$$(SBP0 - SBP1) = b_0 + b_1 Group + e, \qquad (5.8)$$

where *SBP0* and *SBP1* are baseline and follow-up recordings of *SBP*, respectively; b_0 is the intercept; b_1 is the regression coefficient for the treatment group; and *e* is the residual error term. Equation 5.8 illustrates a linear model in which the observed *SBP* reduction (= *SBP0* – *SBP1*) is partitioned into two components: one (represented by b_0) denotes the amount of *SBP* reduction that is common to both groups of patients, and the other (represented by b_1) denotes the differential amount of *SBP* reduction attributable to the effects of the new medication compared to the placebo control group. Group is thus a binary variable denoting the treatment group with the new medication (coded 1) or the placebo control group (reference group, coded 0). The research question is to test whether there is a significant difference in *SBP* reduction between the two groups; that is, whether or not the regression coefficient b_1 is significantly different from zero.

Figure 5.3a shows the DAG for Equation 5.8. There are arrows (directed paths) from *Group* to *SBP0* and *SBP reduction*, but there is no path connecting *SBP0* and *SBP reduction*. The interpretation of Figure 5.3a is that there are differences in baseline *SBP* and changes in *SBP* in the two treatment groups due to receiving different medications. However, the difference in baseline *SBP* is not related to *SBP* reduction. Figure 5.3b is the path diagram for using SEM software packages, such as Amos, to carry out a *t*-test as shown in Equation 5.8. Alternative SEM models are possible for obtaining the same results, but we only present the simplest one. By SEM convention, observed variables are within squares, and the unobserved variable (i.e., measurement errors term *e*) is within circles. In Figure 5.3b, the effect of *Group* on *SBP0* is also estimated, and this does not affect the estimation of the relation between *Group* and *SBP* reduction. If the randomisation is properly implemented, the effect of *Group* on *SBP0* will be small; that is, the average baseline *SBP* is similar in the two treatment groups.

Suppose we now wish to use ANCOVA to carry out the analysis. The regression model for ANCOVA is given as

$$(SBP0 - SBP1) = \beta_0 + \beta_1 Group + \beta_2 SBP0 + \varepsilon, \qquad (5.9)$$

where β_0 is the intercept, β_1 the regression coefficient for *Group*, β_2 the regression coefficient for *SBP0*, and ε the residual error term. *SBP0* is now

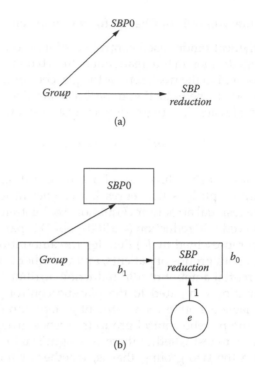

FIGURE 5.3
(a) The directed acyclic graph of the *t*-test for a hypothetical RCT, and (b) the path diagram of the *t*-test for scenario one. In the directed acyclic graph or path diagram, a line with one arrow (→) represents a unidirectional flow of effect from one variable to another. When there is no connecting line between two variables, they are assumed to be independent in the model, so the assumption of the *t*-test is that baseline systolic blood pressure (*SBP0*) does not affect the change in blood pressure (*SBP reduction*).

a covariate; that is, it is considered to influence *SBP* reduction. Figure 5.4a shows the DAG for Equation 5.9. The difference between Figures 5.3a and 5.4a is the arrow from *SBP0* to *SBP reduction*; that is, baseline *SBP* is considered a potential *cause* for the change in *SBP*. To obtain the same results as ANCOVA using SEM, we draw the path diagram in Figure 5.4b. The differences between Figures 5.4b and 5.3b are the addition of the path from *Group* to *SBP0* and the estimation of the residual errors term ε_1.

From the two DAGs and SEM models, it is clear that the difference in results between the *t*-test and ANCOVA is due to the different assumptions adopted in terms of the relation between baseline values and the change from baseline. When choosing different statistical tests, researchers either choose or inadvertently accept different assumptions underpinning these tests. In this example, the difference in results between ANCOVA and the *t*-test is expected to be small because the difference in baseline *SBP* between the two treatment groups is small if randomisation is properly implemented. If, for certain reasons, the difference in the baseline values in the collected

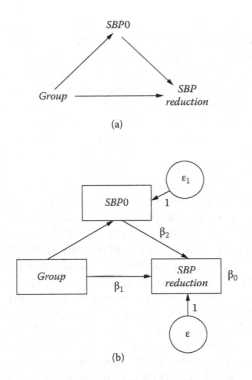

FIGURE 5.4
(a) The directed acyclic graph of the *t*-test for a hypothetical RCT, and (b) the path diagram of the *t*-test for scenario one. Since there is an arrow from *SBP0* to *SBP reduction*, the assumption of ANCOVA is that baseline blood pressure affects change in blood pressure.

sample are large, results from these two methods can be substantially different, giving rise to contradictory interpretations. Nevertheless, if the assumption that there should be no difference between the two groups in the study population holds (as in an RCT), ANCOVA is expected to give a more accurate estimate (Senn 2006).

5.7.2 Scenario Two: The Analysis of Change for Observational Studies

Although RCT is considered the gold standard for study design, its implementation is not always feasible in epidemiological research for reasons such as ethics and high costs. Suppose our hypothetical study is not an RCT but an observational study; for example, patients with baseline $SBP > 180$ mmHg are allocated to the treatment group, and the remaining patients become the control group. These two groups will have different baseline *SBP*, and results from the *t*-test and ANCOVA will become different. The question is, which one, the *t*-test or ANCOVA, gives rise to the correct answer.

Unfortunately, there is no simple solution. When the study groups have not resulted from an effective randomisation process, the validity of the results of analysis following the use of ANCOVA or the *t*-test depends on opposing and inherently untestable assumptions. Many discussions of this phenomenon in the literature are mainly philosophical because both ANCOVA and the *t*-test are well-established and *statistically valid* methods—it is the context of their application and associated interpretation that creates confusion. As explained previously, using the *t*-test implicitly assumes that baseline values will not affect the changes from baseline caused by the interventions (irrespective of whether or not baselines are balanced across groups). Therefore, if the intervention given to one group had no additional effect compared to that given to another group, the post-treatment values would have changed by exactly the same amount, irrespective of baseline values. In contrast, ANCOVA assumes that baseline values will affect the changes from baseline. If the intervention given to one group had no additional effect compared to that given to another group, then differences in the changes from baseline between the two groups would still be observed (Mohr 2000).

Therefore, if the medication has no genuine effect, we should observe no change in *SBP* for both groups; or, its effect on *SBP* is constant irrespective of baseline *SBP* (e.g., 10 mmHg for all patients), so we should observe the same amount of change in *SBP* in both groups. If such assumptions hold, the *t*-test should be the preferred method. On the other hand, if such assumptions do not hold, the *t*-test will give biased results. For instance, due to RTM, as discussed in Chapter 4, people with higher blood pressure at the first reading tend to have lower blood pressure at the second reading due to measurement errors or physiological fluctuations in blood pressure. Therefore, the average blood pressure in the treatment group is likely to become lower even if the medication has no genuine effect. Although this phenomenon of RTM may also occur in the control group, the amount of blood pressure change is likely to be smaller in the control group because its average blood pressure at baseline was not as high as in the treatment group. Therefore, ANCOVA may yield unbiased results by adjusting for baseline blood pressure, and the DAG in Figure 5.5 illustrates why this is possible. There are two paths in Figure 5.5 between *Group* and *SBP reduction*: a direct path: *Group →SBP reduction*, and an indirect path: *Group → SBP0 → RTM → SBP reduction*.

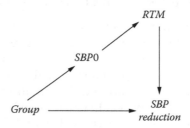

FIGURE 5.5
Directed acyclic graph of ANOVA for scenario two. The adjustment of *SBP0* will block the indirect path from *Group* to *SBP reduction* via *RTM*.

The observed association between *Group* and *SBP reduction* is the sum of the direct and indirect effects. The effect in the direct path is genuine and what we try to estimate, whilst the effect in the indirect path is spurious. When *SBP0* is adjusted for, the indirect path will then be blocked.

Note that the reality in most observational studies is far more complex than the DAG in Figure 5.5, in which the only source of bias is RTM and there is only one baseline covariate to be considered. In most epidemiological studies, there are usually many baseline covariates, and their values in the different subject groups may be unbalanced. For instance, propensity scores estimation has been proposed to overcome the bias caused by the imbalance of baseline covariate values (Rubin 1997; Joffe and Rosenbaum 1999; Luellen et al. 2005). The propensity score of a subject is the probability of that subject being in the treatment group based on the distribution of baseline covariates. Differences in the outcomes between groups may subsequently be estimated based on stratification by the propensity scores, which may be treated as a continuous variable or categorical variable. However, this does not alter the implicit assumption in ANCOVA that the differences in baseline values can cause differences in the changes from baseline due to either RTM or a genuine relationship between changes and initial values. However, if this assumption is incorrect, the adjustment of baseline covariates or propensity scores may exacerbate the bias, rather than eliminate it. A more detailed discussion on the adjustment of baseline values in observational studies can be found in Glymour et al. (2005) and Glymour (2006).

5.8 Conclusion

This chapter demonstrates for the first time that vector geometry can provide simple, intuitive and elegant illustrations of the differences in statistical power amongst three univariate statistical methods commonly adopted in clinical research to analyse data from pre-/post-test study design. It is shown that the commonly accepted concept that ANCOVA is the most powerful method is not strictly correct. Due to the loss of one degree of freedom, ANCOVA might have poorer power than testing post-test scores when the sample size is small and the correlation between pre- and post-test scores is low. This is demonstrated by simulations. Theoretical considerations and simulations show that MANOVA will always have poorer power than ANCOVA, and it is shown for the first time that there is a mathematical relation between the *F*-values of these two methods. Vector geometry also shows that ANCOVA and change scores will give rise to the same estimate of group difference if and only if the pre-test (baseline) values are expected to be balanced. In most epidemiologic studies, this assumption is not tenable, and, therefore, adjustment for baseline values will yield results different from those using simple change scores. Therefore, one needs to be very cautious in using ANCOVA in non-randomised studies, especially when the difference in the baseline value of the adjusted covariate between the exposed/non-exposed groups is caused by the criterion used to select participants in the groups. Failure to recognize this can give rise to Lord's paradox and yield misleading results.

6

Collinearity and Multicollinearity

6.1 Introduction: Problems of Collinearity in Linear Regression

A common problem in the use of multiple regression when analysing clinical and epidemiological data is the occurrence of explanatory variables (covariates) that are not statistically independent; that is, where correlations amongst covariates are not zero (Glantz and Slinker 2001). Most textbooks emphasise that there should be no significant associations between covariates, as this gives rise to the problem known as *collinearity* (Slinker and Glantz 1985; Pedhazur 1997; Chatterjee et al. 2000; Glantz and Slinker 2001; Maddala 2001; Miles and Shelvin 2001). When there are more than two covariates that are correlated, this is *multicollinearity*. Note that the original definition of collinearity and multicollinearity is that at least one covariate can be expressed as a linear combination of the others (Maddala 2001). For example, suppose the statistical model for Y regressed on p covariates X_1, X_2, ..., and X_p is given as

$$Y = b_0 + b_1 X_1 + b_2 X_2 + ... + b_p X_p + e,$$

then collinearity means that at least one covariate X_i can be expressed as

$$X_i = a_0 + a_1 X_1 + a_2 X_2 + ... + a_{i-1} X_{i-1} + a_{i+1} X_{i+1} + ... + a_p X_p.$$

In the literature, this is generally known as *perfect* collinearity or multicollinearity and causes serious problems in computation because the data matrix containing the variances and covariances of all Xs is not full-ranked, and therefore, it is not invertible. Perfect collinearity is generally rare and is often due to mathematical coupling amongst covariates (examples in biomedical research can be found in our previous study [Tu et al. 2005c]). The simplest solution to perfect collinearity is to drop at least one of the collinear covariates.

Collinearity and multicollinearity can seriously distort the interpretation of a regression model. The role of each covariate is to cause increased inaccuracy, as expressed through bias within the regression coefficients (Maddala

2001), and increased uncertainty, as expressed through coefficient standard errors (Slinker and Glantz 1985; Pedhazur 1997; Chatterjee et al. 2000; Glantz and Slinker 2001; Maddala 2001; Miles and Shelvin 2001). Consequently, regression coefficients biased by collinearity might cause variables, which demonstrate no significant relationship with the outcome when considered in isolation, to become highly significant in conjunction with collinear variables, yielding an elevated risk of false-positive results (Type I error). Alternatively, multiple regression coefficients might show no statistical significance due to incorrectly estimated wide confidence intervals, yielding an elevated risk of false-negative results (Type II error).

Mild or moderate collinearity or multicollinearity is not necessarily a serious problem. For instance, statistical adjustment for confounding in epidemiology is to utilize collinearity to nullify the effects of the exposure variables that are mixed with the effect of confounding variables (MacKinnon et al. 2000). However, severe or perfect collinearity/multicollinearity is definitely a serious problem and gives rise to misleading results. Classical examples used by many textbooks to illustrate multicollinearity are those in which several explanatory variables are significantly correlated with the outcome variable using correlation or simple regression. Then, within a multiple regression model, none or few of the covariates are statistically significant, yet the overall variance of the dependent variable explained by the covariates is high (as measured by R^2). This is because the information given by each covariate "overlaps" with other covariates due to multicollinearity. Thus, it becomes hard, if not impossible, to distinguish amongst the individual contributions of each covariate to the outcome variance.

It might be helpful to use Venn diagrams to illustrate the problems of collinearity in a regression model in which Y is regressed on X and Z (Figure 6.1a and 6.1b). Each circle represents the variance of each corresponding variable. The overlapped area is the covariance between two or three variables. For instance, $b + d$ is the covariance between Y and Z. Multiple regression seeks to estimate the *independent* contribution of X and Z to the variance of Y; that is, to estimate a and b for X and Z, respectively. Figure 6.1a shows the scenario where the correlation between X and Z is small; that is, c and d are relatively small compared to a and b. In contrast, Figure 6.1b shows the scenario where the correlation between X and Z is high; that is, c and d are large. Although correlations between Y and X and between Y and Z remain similar, and the total explained variance (a, b, and d) of Y explained by X and Z remain similar, a large correlation between X and Z makes a and b become smaller and statistically non-significant.

The *independent* contribution of one covariate estimated by multiple regression is established by statistically adjusting for other covariates in the same model. As a result, the independent contribution of one covariate is conditional on the choice of covariates 'adjusted for' and will not remain the same when these covariates become different. Furthermore, although multiple regression can estimate an independent contribution of one covariate

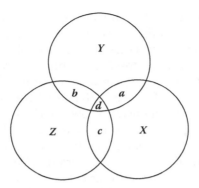

(a) The scenario where the correlation
between X and Z is small.

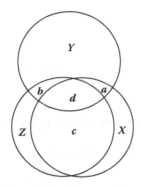

(b) The scenario where the correlation
between X and Z is large.

FIGURE 6.1
Venn diagram for illustration of collinearity. (a) Variables with little collinearity; (b) variable
with large collinearity. *Source*: Figures 1a and 1b with modifications from Tu, Y.K., Kellet, M.,
Clerehugh, V., Gilthorpe, M.S., *British Dental Journal*, 199, pp. 458–461, 2005. With permission.

to the variation of the outcome by statistically adjusting for other covariates, the interpretation of this statistically independent contribution might
be problematic. Suppose b_X is the partial regression coefficient of X when Y
is regressed on X and Z. The correct interpretation is that if all subjects have
the same value of Z (usually it is the mean of Z), when X increases by one
unit, Y will increase by b_X unit. The question should be asked is: is it possible
in reality that all subjects have the same value of Z? It has been shown in
Chapter 5 that Lord's paradox arises when the assumption that all subjects
have the same baseline value is questionable.

An important point often overlooked is that even when regression coefficients remain statistically significant, collinearity and multicollinearity
can cause serious problems in the interpretation of results from a regression

analysis. For instance, the relationship between the outcome and a covariate might be reversed when another covariate is entered into the model. This is also a limitation of using a Venn diagram in the explanation of the problems of collinearity because it is impossible to show the reverse of the relation between outcome and explanatory variables in Venn diagrams. Therefore, in this chapter, following a brief review of the statistical concepts of collinearity and multicollinearity, we demonstrate how vector geometry can provide an intuitive understanding of the problems caused by collinearity in regression analyses, and we use vector geometry to illustrate the limitation of currently proposed solutions to collinearity in the literature. Vector geometry has been occasionally used in some statistical or econometric textbooks (Wonnacott and Wonnacott 1979, 1981; Belsley 1991) to explain the problem of collinearity, such as inflated confidence intervals. However, vector geometry can show how the impact of collinearity is much broader than that currently recognized in the literature.

6.2 Collinearity

Consider a multiple regression model with two covariates:

$$y = b_0 + b_1 x_1 + b_2 x_2 + \varepsilon, \tag{6.1}$$

where y is the outcome, x_1 and x_2 are two covariates, ε is the random error term, b_0 is the intercept, and b_1 and b_2 are the multiple regression coefficients for x_1 and x_2, respectively. The size of b_1 and b_2 will be affected by changing the scales of the covariates, such as using metres instead of millimetres, but the strength of association with the outcome (i.e., the statistical significance) will not be changed. It is therefore appropriate for our illustration to consider the *standardised regression coefficient* of b_1, β_1, because the scale of x_1 does not affect the size of β_1. The standardised regression coefficient is derived from the pairwise correlations of y, x_1 and x_2 (Glantz and Slinker 2001) by

$$\beta_1 = (r_{y1} - r_{12} r_{y2}) / (1 - r_{12}^2), \tag{6.2}$$

where r_{y1} is the correlation between y and x_1, r_{y2} is the correlation between y and x_2, and r_{12} is the correlation between covariates x_1 and x_2.

Assuming that r_{y1} and r_{y2} remain unchanged, whilst r_{12} becomes larger (i.e., there is increasing collinearity between x_1 and x_2), β_1 will become smaller because the numerator in Equation 6.2 will become much smaller even though the denominator is also reduced. For instance, to simplify the scenario, suppose r_{y1} is equal to r_{y2}; that is, both covariates have the same strength of association with the outcome. If r_{12} is zero, $\beta_1 = r_{y1}$, which indicates that the association between y and x_1 is not affect by x_2; similarly, the association between y and x_2 is not affect by x_1. This is because x_1 and x_2 are independent since their correlation is zero. If r_{12} is now 0.1, $\beta_1 = 0.91r_{y1}$; if r_{12} increases to 0.5, $\beta_1 = 0.67r_{y1}$; and if r_{12} increases to 0.8, $\beta_1 = 0.56r_{y1}$. Thus, the size of the association between y and x_1 is affected by the increasing correlation between x_1 and x_2.

A major concern within collinearity is what happens to the standard error of b_1, denoted S_{b_1}, given as (Glantz and Slinker 2001)

$$S_{b_1} = \sqrt{\frac{MS_{res}}{\sum (x_1 - \overline{x}_1)^2 (1 - r_{12}^2)}}, \qquad (6.3)$$

where MS_{res} is the residual mean squared error. In a model with only two covariates, as here, this is $MS_{res} = SS_{res}/(n-3)$ where n is the sample size and SS_{res} is the residual sum of squares (i.e., the unexplained variance of y). In Equation 6.3, if r_{12} is large (irrespective of sign), then $1 - r_{12}^2$ is close to zero, and hence S_{b_1} will be increased. Thus, the standard error of b_1 and the associated confidence interval it gives rise to will be inflated. Similarly, the same applies to the second (correlated) covariate, x_2. Consequently, significance testing of both x_1 and x_1 is substantially affected by the correlation between them. Moreover, as r_{12} approaches unity, simultaneous estimation of both covariates will become impossible as S_{b_1} becomes infinite, and one covariate would need to be removed from the regression model in order to attain a computable regression model. This situation is known as *perfect collinearity*.

6.3 Multicollinearity

In a multiple regression with k covariates ($k > 2$),

$$y = b_0 + b_1 x_1 + b_2 x_2 + \ldots + b_k x_k + \varepsilon, \qquad (6.4)$$

the standard error of covariate b_i, S_{bi}, is given

$$S_{bi} = \sqrt{\frac{MS_{res}}{\sum (x_i - \overline{x}_i)^2 (1 - R_i^2)}}, \qquad (6.5)$$

where R_i^2 is the square of the multiple correlation coefficient for x_i regressed on all remaining covariates, which effectively shows how much of the variation in x_i can be explained by the other covariates. Thus, R_i^2 is a measure of the association between x_i and the other covariates. If R_i^2 is zero, x_i is independent of all other covariates. However, if R_i^2 is large, most of the variation in x_i can be explained by the remaining covariates in the regression model.

To diagnose multicollinearity in multiple regression, one might use the variance inflation factor (VIF), which is incorporated into mainstream statistical software packages and defined by (Slinker and Glantz 1985; Pedhazur 1997; Chatterjee et al. 2000; Glantz and Slinker 2001; Maddala 2001; Miles and Shelvin 2001)

$$VIF = \frac{1}{1 - R_i^2}. \tag{6.6}$$

Many textbooks suggest that if the VIF is more than 10, there is a serious collinearity problem (Slinker and Glantz 1985; Pedhazur 1997; Chatterjee et al. 2000; Glantz and Slinker 2001; Maddala 2001; Miles and Shelvin 2001). However, multicollinearity does not necessarily require large correlations amongst covariates for this value to be achieved. For instance, consider x_1, x_2 and x_3 to be independent and to have equal variances (hence r_{12}, r_{23} and r_{13} are all zero) and define a fourth variable such that $x_4 = x_1 + x_2 + x_3$. It can be shown that, in this instance, $R_i^2 = 1$ for each of the four covariates because any one of the four variables can be derived mathematically from the remaining three. Consequently, there is perfect multicollinearity amongst the four variables, yet the pairwise correlations between x_4 and x_1, x_2 or x_3 do not exceed $0.58 (= 1/\sqrt{3})$:

$$corr(x_4, x_1) = \frac{Cov(x_4, x_1)}{\sqrt{Var(x_4)Var(x_1)}} = \frac{Var(x_1)}{\sqrt{Var(x_1)(Var(x_1) + Var(x_2) + Var(x_3))}} = \frac{1}{\sqrt{3}}.$$

An example within periodontal research is, again, where the clinical attachment level (CAL) is derived from the sum of probing pocket depth (PPD) and gingival recession (GR). If all the three variables were entered simultaneously in a regression model, either no solution could be obtained or the computer software would give a warning because the data matrix could not be inverted to obtain a solution for the regression equation, and one of the covariates would need to be dropped. If the procedure of variable selection were automatic, such as forward or backward stepwise selection (Miller 2002), only two of the covariates would be retained, and the computer algorithm could never select the third. However, which two covariates should be selected as the more relevant/important is not a decision to be made by the computer. The problem of collinearity or multicollinearity is not solved by computer software simply because one of the collinear variables will be automatically dropped (backward stepwise) or never selected (forward stepwise). Statistical modelling of clinical data should be based upon a sound theoretical under-standing or hypothesis of the biological system under investigation, not com-puter algorithms. The decision whether or not a variable should be entered (or removed) should be made by the researchers based on *a priori* biologi-cal and clinical knowledge. In circumstances of perfect collinearity (as with PD, CAL, and GR), the researcher is responsible, in the context of the model being developed, for the decision over which clinical variables provide no additional information pertaining to the outcome when there is redundancy amongst the variables. Moreover, if perfectly collinear explanatory variables suffer measurement error, thereby masking a perfect inter-relationship, none might be removed by the computer software automatically because it can still proceed with the mathematical calculations, albeit only because of the presence of measurement error.

6.4 Mathematical Coupling and Collinearity

Within multiple regression, if one covariate can be algebraically derived from the remaining covariates, collinearity or multicollinearity is an inevitable problem as there will potentially be large correlations amongst all function-ally related variables due to mathematical coupling (Archie 1981; Andersen 1990). Moreover, perfect collinearity or multicollinearity will render the inter-pretation of the regression model as misleading. Regrettably, many clinical variables are either mathematically related to others (as with PPD, GR and CAL) or different biomarkers for the same diseases, for example, insulin and blood sugar for diabetes. Therefore, problems due to collinearity or multi-collinearity may cause difficulties in the meaningful interpretation of results from studies that suffer these problems.

6.5 Vector Geometry of Collinearity

In n-dimensional vector geometry, collinearity and multicollinearity imply that the angles between the collinear vectors are very small. In other words, the directions of these vectors are nearly parallel. For perfect collinearity between two variables, the two corresponding vectors are parallel and over-lapped (if in the same direction, the correlation is 1, or if in the opposite direc-tion, the correlation is –1); the only difference is the *length* of the vectors.

As explained in Chapter 2, to regress y on x and z simultaneously is to find the orthogonal projection of the vector y onto the plane spanned by

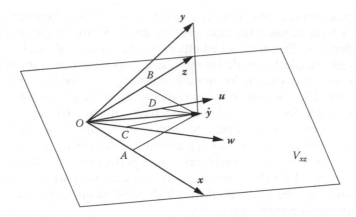

FIGURE 6.2
Vector geometry of collinearity. As x and z span the same subspace (V_{xz}) as u and w, the projection of y on V_{xz}, $\hat{y} = \overline{OA} * x + \overline{OB} * z = \overline{OC} * w + \overline{OD} * u$. The partial regression coefficients for w ($\overline{OC}/\|x\|$) and u ($\overline{OD}/\|z\|$) are smaller than those for x ($\overline{OA}/\|x\|$) and z ($\overline{OB}/\|z\|$).

vectors x and z, and then to use the parallelogram rule to find the weights for x and z to portray the projected vector $\hat{y}$. For instance, in Figure 6.2, $\hat{y} = \overline{OA} * x + \overline{OB} * z$, where $\overline{OA}/\|x\|$ and $\overline{OB}/\|z\|$ are the partial regression coefficients for x and z, respectively. Suppose y is now regressed on u and w, and the correlation between u and w is greater than that between x and z. Although vectors u and w span the same space as x and z, and $\hat{y}$ is unchanged (Figure 6.2), the partial regression coefficients for w ($\overline{OC}/\|x\|$) and u ($\overline{OD}/\|z\|$) are smaller than those for x ($\overline{OA}/\|x\|$) and z ($\overline{OB}/\|z\|$). Therefore, although the two regression models explain the same amount of variance of y, x and z might be statistically significant, whereas w and u might not be. Then, one might gain an impression that x and z are important explanatory variables for y, but w and u are not.

6.5.1 Reversed Relation between the Outcome and Covariate due to Collinearity

An important symptom of collinearity and multicollinearity, useful in the diagnosis of collinearity, is that the direction of the association between the covariate and the outcome is reversed after adjustment for other covariates. It is easily shown in vector geometry why and when this occurs (Figure 6.3). When the correlation between covariates is large, and the angle between the collinear vectors is thus very small, the projection of y might fall on the *outside* of the two vectors on the plane spanned by the collinear variable vectors. The direction of the association for the covariate vector that has the greater correlation with the outcome will remain unchanged, whereas the direction of the other covariate vector will be reversed. Sometimes, the reversed relation might still be statistically significant. Therefore, the significance or the extent

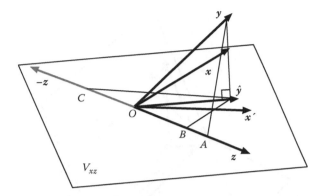

FIGURE 6.3
Vector geometry of a reversed relation between the outcome y and the covariate z after adjustment for x. In simple regression, where y is regressed on z, the regression coefficient for z $(\overline{OA}/\|z\|)$ is positive (because $\overline{OA}$ is in the same direction of z). In multiple regression, where y is regressed on x and z, the sign of the regression coefficient for z $(\overline{OB}/\|z\|)$ is still positive (because $\overline{OB}$ is in the same direction of z). However, when y is regressed on x' and z, the relation between y and z can be reversed where x' is highly correlated with z because the partial regression coefficient for z $(\overline{OC}/\|z\|)$ is in the opposite direction of z.

of significance (or the absence of significance) of covariates cannot be used as a key criterion in the diagnosis of collinearity in a regression model.

6.5.2 Unstable Regression Models due to Collinearity

Another serious consequence of multicollinearity is that a slight modification of the data might induce substantial changes in the results of the regression analysis in terms of the direction of association and model fit (R^2). For instance, a regression model might achieve a large R^2 in one data set but attain a very small R^2 using a slightly modified or subtly different data set; or the relation between the outcome and covariates is substantially different between one subset and another, where both subsets are randomly selected from the same original data. When y is regressed on x and z, $\hat{y}_{xz}$ is the projection of y on the V_{xz} plane within vector geometry. The proportion of variance of y explained by x and z is $(\|\hat{y}_{xz}\|/\|y\|)^2$. Figure 6.4 shows that the projection of y ($\hat{y}_{xz}$) is closer to x, and therefore the regression coefficient is positive for x and negative for z. However, suppose the same study is repeated by sampling different subjects from the same population. The new x (x') and new z (z') will be highly correlated with the x and z, respectively, and therefore the correlation between y and x' or between y and z' is probably similar to that between y and x or between y and z, respectively. However, the multiple regression coefficients for x' and z' can substantially differ from those for x and z. From a geometrical viewpoint, the angle between x and z is very small, and therefore the inclination of the plane spanned by x and z in a three-dimensional space can be altered considerably with only slight

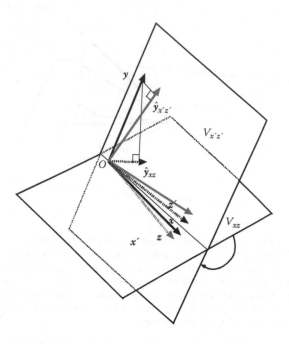

FIGURE 6.4

Vector geometry of unstable regression due to collinearity. When y is regressed on x and z, $\hat{y}_{xz}$ is the projection of y on the V_{xz} plane. The proportion of variance of y explained by x and z is $(\|\hat{y}_{xz}\|/\|y\|)^2$. As $\hat{y}_{xz}$ is on the 'outside' (as explained in Figure 6.3) and x is closer to $\hat{y}_{xz}$ than z, the partial regression coefficient for x will be positive, and that for z will be negative. When the same study is repeated by sampling different subjects from the same population, the new x (x') and new z (z') will be highly correlated with x and z, respectively. However, the inclination of the V_{xz} plane can be substantially different from the inclination of the $V_{x'z'}$ plane. In the figure, the $V_{x'z'}$ plane is a 120° rotation of the V_{xz} plane, and the length of projection of y ($\hat{y}_{x'z'}$) on the $V_{x'z'}$ the plane becomes much greater than $\hat{y}_{xz}$. Moreover, z' now is closer to $\hat{y}_{x'z'}$, and therefore, the regression coefficient for z' will now be positive, whilst that for x' will now be negative.

changes in x and z. In other words, the relation between y and the V_{xz} plane is relatively unstable when the angle between vectors x and z is small; that is, when collinearity is severe. Figure 6.4 shows that slight changes in the positions of x and z in three-dimensional space might cause a rotation of the V_{xz} plane and dramatically change the direction of associations between the outcome and the collinear covariates.

6.5.3 The Relation between the Outcome–Explanatory Variable's Correlations and Collinearity

Traditional diagnostics of collinearity, such as VIF or conditional index, concentrate on the correlation structure between explanatory variables and totally overlook the correlation between the outcome and covariates.

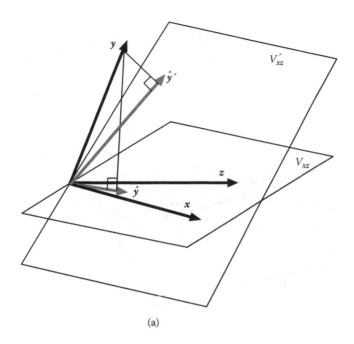

(a)

FIGURE 6.5
Vector geometry of the relation between collinearity and the outcome-covariate correlations.
(a) When the correlation between variables y and both x and z are weak, small changes in the
plane spanned by x and z caused by sampling variations might cause substantial differences
in the partial regression coefficients. The length of the projection of y onto plane V_{xz} ($\hat{y}$) is much
shorter than that of the projection on V'_{xz} ($\hat{y}'$). (b) In contrast, when the correlations between y
and both x and z is strong, small changes in the plane spanned by x and z (caused by sampling
variations) could cause small differences in the partial regression coefficients. The length of
the projection of y onto plane V_{xz} ($\hat{y}$) is similar to that of the projection on V'_{xz} ($\hat{y}'$).

However, vector geometry provides a unique insight to the problem of collinearity. Figure 6.5 shows that when the correlation between the outcome
y and the covariates x and z is small, the same regression model applied
to different data might yield substantial variation in the multiple correlation (R) (or R^2, as it is most often presented) and regression coefficients. In
contrast, when the correlation between the outcome y and the covariates x
and z is strong, the same regression model applied to different data yields
smaller differences in the multiple correlation (or R^2) and regression coefficients. Therefore, the impact of collinearity should also take into consideration the correlations between the outcome and all covariates. For any
subgroup of covariates in one data set, the VIF and the conditional index
will always be the same, yet the problem of collinearity might vary from
one outcome to another.

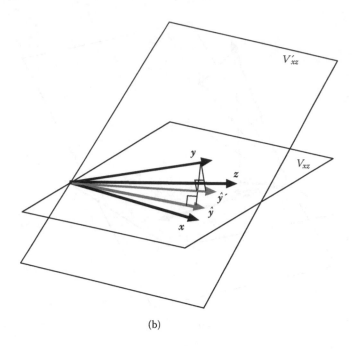

(b)

FIGURE 6.5 (continued).

6.6 Geometrical Illustration of Principal Components Analysis as a Solution to Multicollinearity

Principal component analysis (PCA) is one of several 'solutions' to the problem of multicollinearity that can be found in the statistical literature (Slinker and Glantz 1985; Chatterjee et al. 2000; Glantz and Slinker 2001; Maddala 2001; Miles and Shelvin 2001). The pros and cons of using PCA have been discussed in great detail in the literature. A potential caveat of PCA, as pointed out by Hadi and Ling (1998), can be elegantly illustrated by vector geometry.

The basic concept underlining PCA is to decompose the collinear explanatory variables (usually standardised) into several orthogonal (i.e., uncorrelated) components, where the number of principal components is equal to the number of explanatory variables. These principal components are ordered according to the proportion of variation in the correlation matrix **X** containing all the explanatory variables. As these components are deliberately generated to be orthogonal, there will be no problem of collinearity in the subsequent regression analyses. In practice, researchers usually regress the outcome on the first few components that explain most of the variation in **X**.

The scree plot, which plots the eigenvalues (corresponding to the extent of variation in **X** explained by each principal component) against the number of principal components, is the most often used method to determine the number of principal components to be used in the regression model (Slinker and Glantz 1985; Chatterjee et al. 2000). The problem with this approach is that, although the (principal) components selected explain most of the variation in **X**, there is no guarantee that these components explain most of the *outcome* variance (Hadi and Ling 1998). The worst case scenario is that, of a total k possible principal components (i.e., when there are exactly k covariates), the first $k - 1$ might explain little in the outcome variable, and the last principal component alone (that is perhaps to be discarded) contributes almost everything to the outcome variation.

Although detailed mathematical treatments of this paradoxical phenomenon using matrix algebra can be found in Hadi and Ling (1998) and Cuadras (1998), vector geometry can provide a simple intuitive illustration. Figure 6.6 uses the outcome variable y and two explanatory variables x and z to show how this phenomenon occurs. When the vector of y, **y**, falls on the outside of x and z, the second principal component might have a greater correlation with y than the first principal component. Figure 6.7 uses the outcome variable y and three explanatory variables x, z and w to show how this phenomenon occurs. Although we need four dimensions to illustrate the relation between y and x, z and w, we only need three dimensions to illustrate the relation between the projection of y, $\hat{y}$, in the space spanned by the three explanatory variables. In Figure 6.7, the third principal component is correlated with $\hat{y}$, but, in contrast, the first and second principal components are nearly orthogonal to $\hat{y}$, and therefore nearly orthogonal to y. A similar geometric approach can be found in Wonnacott and Wonnacott (1979, 1981), but in their figure they showed y instead of $\hat{y}$. As a result, their figure becomes a little unrealistic because if y and three principal components only span a three-dimensional space, this implies that the variance of y can be completely explained by the three explanatory variables.

Where our discussion is applied to k explanatory variables, it is possible that the first $k - 1$ principal components are nearly orthogonal to y, whilst the kth principal component (which is perhaps to be discarded) is correlated with y.

6.7 Example: Mineral Loss in Patients Receiving Parenteral Nutrition

In this section we use a data set from Table D-5, Appendix D, in the textbook on multiple regression by Glantz and Slinker (2001) on mineral loss in

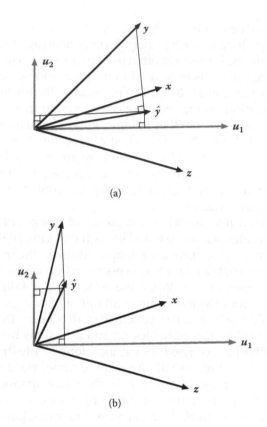

(a)

(b)

FIGURE 6.6
Vector geometry of the use of principal component analysis (PCA) as a solution to multicollinearity: two explanatory variables. (a) The first principal component (PC_1) not only explains
more variation in the covariance or correlation matrix X for x and z than the second principal
component (PC_2) but it also explains more variance of y than PC_2. The vector for PC_1 is u_1,
and the vector for PC_2 is u_2. (b) It is possible that, although PC_1 explains more variation in the
covariance or correlation matrix X for x and z than PC_2, PC_1 may be nearly orthogonal to $\hat{y}$, the
projection of y, on the space spanned by x and z.

patients receiving parenteral nutrition (Lipkin et al. 1988). It is a very good
introductory book on regression analysis for medical and epidemiological
researchers. As explained in Glantz and Slinker (2001), hospitalised patients
who are not able to eat normally must be given intravenous nutrients, a process called parenteral nutrition. However, it is noted that this process leads
to significant cariuresis; that is, loss of calcium via the urine. The degree
of urine calcium loss varies considerably, but sometimes this loss is greater
than what has been given in the intravenous fluid. Therefore, some of the
lost calcium comes from the bones, which play a vital role in maintaining the
balance of calcium in the blood. Cariuresis can be affected by the composi-
tion of parenteral nutrition solutions. Urinary calcium excretion is related to

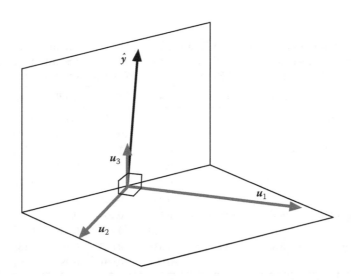

FIGURE 6.7
Vector geometry of the use of PCA as a solution to multicollinearity: three explanatory variables. The projection of y ($\hat{y}$) is nearly orthogonal to the plane spanned by vectors of PC_1 (u_1) and PC_2 (u_2). Therefore, $\hat{y}$ is only correlated with u_3; that is, y is highly correlated with PC_3 but weakly correlated with PC_1 and PC_2.

intravenous calcium intake and other ions such as phosphates in the intravenous fluids (Lipkin et al. 1988).

Urinary calciums (Ca_U), dietary calciums (Ca_D), dietary protein level (P_D), urinary sodium (Na_U) and glomerular filtration rates (GFR; glomeruli are small intertwined loops in the kidney responsible for production of urine, and GFR is an indicator of kidney function) are measured, and the aim of statistical analysis is to investigate the relationship between Ca_U and the other four variables. We first take a look at the bivariate correlations amongst all five variables (Table 6.1): the level of urinary calciums (Ca_U) is positively associated with the four explanatory variables (covariates) and most strongly correlated with dietary calciums (Ca_D). Amongst the four covariates, Ca_D is highly correlated with P_D ($r = 0.882$), and GFR is highly correlated with Na_U ($r = 0.616$).

We first run a multiple linear regression, and the results are shown in Table 6.2. Whilst Ca_D, GFR and Na_U all have positive associations with the level of urinary calciums, there is a negative relation between Ca_U and P_D. Although this negative regression coefficient (–0.51) is not statistically significant, it is contradictory to the positive correlation between Ca_U and P_D we observe in Table 6.1. Can we therefore conclude, based on the results in Table 6.2, that the level of dietary proteins is not associated with excretion of calciums in urine after adjusting for the level of dietary calciums, urinary sodiums and GFR?

TABLE 6.1

Pearson Correlations between the Five Variables, Urinary Calciums (Ca_U), Dietary Calciums (Ca_D), Dietary Protein Level (P_D), Urinary Sodium (Na_U) and Glomerular Filtration Rates (GFR) in 27 Patients Receiving Intravenous Nutrition

	Mean	SD		Ca_U	Ca_D	GFR	Na_U	P_D
Ca_U (mg/12 h)	74.67	61.12	r	1	0.758	0.410	0.493	0.634
			p		<0.001	0.034	0.009	<0.001
Ca_D (mg/12 h)	173.04	160.69	r	0.758	1	0.161	0.164	0.882
			p	<0.001		0.421	0.414	<0.001
GFR (mL/min)	50.22	17.66	r	0.410	0.161	1	0.616	0.212
			p	0.034	0.421		0.001	0.288
Na_U (meq/12 h)	36.15	38.58	r	0.493	0.164	0.616	1	0.183
			p	0.009	0.414	0.001		0.362
P_D (g/day)	36.63	29.83	r	0.634	0.882	0.212	0.183	1
			p	<0.001	<0.001	0.288	0.362	

Note: SD: standard deviation; *r*: Pearson correlation; *p*: p-value. meq: milliequivalents.

TABLE 6.2

Multiple Linear Regression for Urinary Calciums (Ca_U) as the Outcome and Dietary Calciums (Ca_D), Dietary Protein Level (P_D), Urinary Sodium (Na_U) and Glomerular Filtration Rates (GFR) as Covariates

	Coefficients	SE	*t*	*p*-value	Beta
Ca_D	0.35	0.09	3.88	0.00	0.91
GFR	0.43	0.49	0.88	0.39	0.12
Na_U	0.50	0.22	2.25	0.04	0.31
P_D	−0.51	0.48	−1.06	0.30	−0.25

Note: SE: standard errors; Beta: standardised regression coefficients.

The concern here is with the correlations amongst covariates, especially between Ca_D and P_D ($r = 0.882$). As nutrition rich in protein is also rich in calcium, it becomes difficult to differentiate their independent contribution to the excretion of calcium in urine. Consequently, whilst P_D has the second highest positive correlation with Ca_U, it turns out to have a non-significant negative regression coefficient in multiple regression. Although the change in the direction of relationship between Ca_U and P_D might indicate a serious problem of collinearity, the VIF is only 4.5 for Ca_D, 4.6 for P_D and 1.6 for GFR and Na_U. As a result, Glantz and Slinker (2001) did not consider collinearity a serious problem in this regression model (p. 885). Nevertheless, as we have explained in the previous sections, the change in sign is an indicator of collinearity, and the interpretation of results in Table 6.2 merits caution.

6.8 Solutions to Collinearity

No instant and quick solutions can be universally applied to resolve the collinearity problems illustrated in this chapter because statistical modelling strategies are tailored to specific research questions. However, as shown by our example, where researchers have more of an understanding of the statistical tools they used, the mistake made could have been avoided simply by removing one of the collinear variables.

6.8.1 Removal of Redundant Explanatory Variables

The problems of collinearity and multicollinearity might be diagnosed using either the *VIF* or the *condition index*. Although *VIF* > 10 is the criterion most often suggested by textbooks, this is not the only criterion to be used. The unexpected direction of associations between the outcome and explanatory variables is an important sign of collinearity and multicollinearity. When the direction of association differs between simple correlation/regression and multivariable regression, this does not necessarily indicate that the research has found intriguing results. On the contrary, researchers should carefully examine the relationships amongst all the explanatory variables in the regression model. If some of the collinear variables are redundant in terms of providing no extra useful information, or are simply duplicate measurements of the same variable, the solution is to remove these variables from the model. However, it is not always straightforward to determine which variable or variables are redundant. For instance, in our previous example on parenteral patients, are GFR and P_D redundant and therefore to be removed because they have non-significant associations with Ca_U? From a statistical point of view, they may be considered redundant, as their inclusion in the model does not substantially increase the model R^2. However, this statistical redundancy should not be interpreted as biological redundancy. For example, the non-significant relation between Ca_U and GFR does not necessarily mean that kidney function is not related to the excretion of calcium or that when the content of protein in the intravenous nutrition supply is reduced, the excretion of calcium will not be affected.

6.8.2 Centring

Multicollinearity can be a problem for a covariate when included in a model along with its quadratic form in a non-linear regression, or when also included through a product-interaction term with another variable. For instance, if the research question is whether or not the number of cigarettes smoked and the amount of alcohol consumed have a synergistic effect on the risk of oral cancer, a product term—*smoking-alcohol*—might be generated and entered as an additional covariate, along with *smoking* and *alcohol*. This additional covariate is created by multiplying the *smoking* variable (the number of cigarettes smoked) and the *alcohol* variable (the number of alcoholic units consumed). As *smoking-alcohol* is derived mathematically from both *smoking* and *alcohol*, there will be substantial correlations amongst the three variables. However, the correlation between *smoking-alcohol* and either *smoking* or *alcohol* could be considerably reduced if the interaction term *smoking-alcohol* was generated after the values of *smoking* and *alcohol* were centred (Slinker and Glantz 1985); that is, transformed by subtracting the mean values of each from the original variables. For example, suppose there are five patients in a study, and the number of cigarettes smoked per day by each patient is 5, 10, 15, 20, and 25, respectively. After centring, the values of the variable smoking become –10, –5, 0, 5 and 10 since the mean number of cigarettes smoked is 15.

Apart from problems caused by quadratic terms and product-interaction terms, the centring of explanatory variables, in general, does not solve the problem of collinearity or multicollinearity because, mathematically, the correlation coefficient can be interpreted as a product term of two centred variables divided by their variances. Thus, unless the problem is caused by collinearity/multicollinearity between only the intercept and other explanatory variables, both the direction of association between the outcome and collinear covariates and all associated significance testing remain unchanged after centring collinear covariates. Nevertheless, centring will also change the interpretation of the intercept in the regression model, and as discussed in Chapter 4, centring of certain variables will also affect the estimation of random effects in a multilevel and latent growth curve model.

6.8.3 Principal Component Analysis

PCA has been proposed as a solution to the numerical problems caused by collinearity and multicollinearity (Glantz and Slinker 2001; Slinker and Glantz 1985; Chatterjee et al. 2000). The explanatory variables are standardised and reorganised into uncorrelated components using a mathematical technique known as diagonalisation of a matrix to extract eigenvectors and eigenvalues for the data matrix. Each principal component is a linear combination of all explanatory variables, and the number of principal components is equivalent to the number of explanatory variables. Researchers then usually select the first few principal components that explain most of the variance of the covariates and use multiple regression analysis to regress the outcome on the selected principal components. The regression coefficients of each original explanatory variable are derived from the regression coefficients of the selected principal components. The advantage of PCA is that, by selecting only a few principal components (i.e., not all), the problem of wrong signs amongst regression coefficients (i.e., the sign of regression coefficient being contradictory to expectation) will usually be corrected.

For instance, if we applied PCA to the example in Section 6.8, the eigenvectors for the four principal components are

Variables	Component			
	1	2	3	4
Ca_D	0.573	−0.420	0.049	0.702
GFR	0.409	0.575	−0.707	0.060
Na_U	0.400	0.585	0.705	−0.025
P_D	0.587	−0.388	−0.036	−0.710
Eigenvalue	2.13	1.37	0.36	0.12
Variability (%)	53.3	34.1	9.6	2.9
Cumulative %	53.3	87.5	97.1	100.0

Ca_D and P_D have similar large weights (i.e., large values in the first eigenvector) in the first principal component, whilst GFR and NaU have large positive weights in the second component. The first two components explain 87.5% of variance of the four variables, so we may discard the remaining two components. To undertake principal component regression, we first standardised the four explanatory variables; that is, the means of the four covariates are subtracted from their individual values and they are then divided by their standard deviations. As a result, the transformed four covariates have a mean of zero and unit standard deviation. The principal components are weighted composites of transformed explanatory variables. For example, the first principal component is the weighted composite of the four standardised variables. The weights are given by the first eigenvector, and the variance of *PC1* is 2.13; that is, the first eigenvalue. Following the same procedure, we can derive the other three principal components.

One important drawback of PCA is that the principal components selected might well explain the variances of the covariates but poorly explain the variance of the outcome (Chatterjee et al. 2000; Hadi and Ling 1998) as shown in Figure 6.6. Although PCA is recommended as a solution to collinearity, its usefulness is limited. For instance, when Ca_U is regressed on the four principal components, the proportion of variance in Ca_U explained by each component is just the squares of the standardised regression coefficients, as the four principal components are uncorrelated. Table 6.3 shows the results from multiple regression, where the standardised Ca_U are regressed to the four principal components. Although the first principal component explains the greatest proportion ($0.80^2 = 64\%$) of variance in Ca_U, the fourth principal component explains a greater proportion ($−0.28^2 = 7.8\%$) of variance in Ca_U than the second ($−0.03^2 = 0.09\%$) and third ($−0.12^2 = 0.14\%$) components. The standardised PCA regression coefficients for the four covariates are the multiples of regression coefficient for the principal components and the weights for each of the four original covariates. The regression coefficient for *PC1* in

TABLE 6.3

Results From Multiple Regression With Ca_U Regressed
on the Four Principal Components

	Coefficients	SE	*P*-value	Beta
Principal Component 1	0.55	0.08	<0.001	0.80
Principal Component 2	−0.03	0.09	0.754	−0.03
Principal Component 3	−0.19	0.18	0.299	−0.12
Principal Component 4	−0.81	0.32	0.019	−0.28

Note: SE: standard errors; Beta: standardised regression coefficients.

Table 6.3 is 0.55, so the standardised principal component regression coefficients for Ca_D, GFR, Na_U and P_D are

$$Ca_U = 0.55 * PC1$$

$$= 0.55 * (0.573Ca_D + 0.409GFR + 0.4Na_U + 0.587P_D)$$

$$= 0.315 + 0.225GFR + 0.220Na_U + 0.323P_D$$

Those regression coefficients are quite different from those reported in the column of *Beta* in Table 6.2 but have the same signs as the bivariate correlations in Table 6.1.

An alternative method but related to principal component regression is partial least squares (PLS) regression. Whilst the aim of PCA is to maximise the variance of extracted components extracted consecutively, the aim of PLS is to maximise the covariance between the outcome and components extracted consecutively. Therefore, PLS overcomes the potential limitation of principal component regression, as the first PLS component will always have greater covariance with the outcomes than the other components. Table 6.4 shows the results from PLS and PCA regression with the first component. Whilst the difference in R^2 between the two models is negligible, there are small differences in the regression coefficients. It should be noted that when

TABLE 6.4

Results From PCA Regression and PLS Regression
With the First Component

	PCA		PLS	
	Coefficients	Beta	Coefficients	Beta
Ca_D	0.120	0.315	0.137	0.359
GFR	0.777	0.225	0.672	0.194
Na_U	0.348	0.220	0.370	0.234
P_D	0.661	0.323	0.615	0.300
R^2		64.4%		65.8%

all four components are used as covariates, results from PCA, PLS and OLS will be equivalent, so in practice, only a few components will be retained for the regression analysis. We shall discuss the details about the theory and practice of PLS regression in Chapter 10.

6.8.4 Ridge Regression

Another commonly recommended method by statistical textbooks, though relatively unknown to most epidemiologists and clinicians, is *ridge regression* (Hoerl and Rennard, 1970). The basic concept of ridge regression is that all explanatory variables are standardised to have a mean of zero and a standard deviation of one, and the value k is added to the original data to modify the explanatory variables (Hoerl and Rennard 1970; Chatterjee et al. 2000; Hastie et al., 2009). Usually, k starts from a very small value, such as 0.0001, and gradually increases to, say, 1, and a value of k is selected when the changes in the regression coefficients becomes stable.

More formally, ridge regression is to minimise a penalised residual sum of squares (RSS) in a regression with p covariates:

$$RSS_{ridge}(\beta_j) = \sum_{i=1}^{n}(y_i - \hat{y})^2 + \lambda \sum_{j=1}^{p}\beta_j^2.$$

It can be show that the ridge regression coefficients $\hat{\beta}^{ridge}$ are then given by

$$\hat{\beta}^{ridge} = (\mathbf{X}^{\mathsf{T}}\mathbf{X} + \lambda\mathbf{I})^{-1}\mathbf{X}^{\mathsf{T}}\mathbf{y}.$$

There are a few criteria given in textbooks on how to determine the most appropriate λ. Note that when λ is large enough, all the regression coefficients become zero. Chatterjee et al (2006) provides an accessible explanation of this technique for non-statisticians, and a more technical account can be found in Hastie et al. (2009). One limitation of its use in epidemiological research is that the procedure of ridge regression is not readily available in some standard popular statistical software. Whilst this problem may have been overcome in recent years (e.g., there is a user-written command rx.ridge in Stata), the main problem is that ridge regression is a pure mathematical technique; that is, the solution it provides is essentially to resolve the mathematical computation problem and sometimes has no relevance to substantive research questions. For instance, we applied ridge regression to the cariuresis example data, and Figure 6.8 is the ridge trace plot, which shows traces for the changes in all the four regression coefficients when λ increases from 0 to 100. The analysis was carried out using lm.ridge in package MASS for the statistical software R, and $\lambda = 0.9$ was chosen by the automatic method generalized cross-validation (GCV). The four regression coefficients for Ca_d,

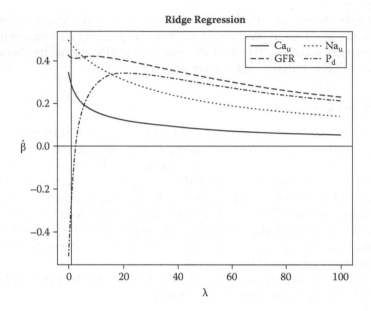

FIGURE 6.8
Ridge trace plot for Cariuresis data. Generalized cross-validation suggests trace $\lambda = 0.9$ is appropriate, but the trace plot seems to suggest that when $\lambda = 20$, the regression coefficients start to become more stable.

GFR, Na_u and P_d at $\lambda = 0.9$ were 0.29, 0.42, 0.48, and -0.26, respectively. These results may have relatively lower residual errors but are still hard to interpret just like the results from OLS regression because of the negative coefficient for P_d. Amongst the four covariates in Figure 6.8, P_d is the one showing the greatest change when λ changes. When λ is zero, it is just as for OLS regression; when λ increases, the coefficients for P_d become less negative and then turns positive when λ is around 3. The coefficient for P_d reaches its maximum when λ is around 20, where the regression coefficients Ca_d, GFR, Na_u and P_d are 0.12, 0.40, 0.31, and 0.34, respectively. Compared to results from PCA and PLS regression, these coefficients are smaller but with the same sign. This example demonstrates the practical difficulty in the application of ridge regression, and this may explain why it is seldom used in epidemiology.

6.9 Conclusion

This chapter illustrates that vector geometry can provide an intuitive understanding of the problems behind collinearity and multicollinearity. Vector geometry can also be a very useful tool to explore the potential impact on the results of linear regression modelling or, in general, statistical adjustment in regression analyses. In clinical and epidemiological research, where most explanatory variables are correlated, the problems of collinearity and multicollinearity may be too frequently overlooked or underestimated due to the lack of an adequate understanding of the consequences of multicollinearity.

Moreover, vector geometry indicates that the current diagnostic tools of collinearity/multicollinearity, such as VIF or the conditional index, may be insufficient or even inadequate. These diagnostic methods mainly focus on the correlations amongst covariates without taking into consideration the correlations between the outcome and all covariates. Collinearity might not be a serious problem in one regression model, yet it might cause misleading results in another where two different outcomes are regressed on the same covariates. Therefore, a new index needs to be developed to measure the severity of collinearity by taking into account the correlations between the outcome and all covariates simultaneously. As pointed out by Hadi and Ling (1998) and illustrated in this chapter using vector geometry, any solution to the problem of multicollinearity should take into consideration the relation between the outcome and its covariates.

7

Is 'Reversal Paradox' a Paradox?

7.1 A Plethora of Paradoxes: The Reversal Paradox

Within the field of probability and statistical science, the *reversal paradox* is best known for categorical variables as *Yule's paradox* or *Simpson's paradox*. This is because George U. Yule noticed this phenomenon as early as 1903 (Yule 1903) when he referred to a paper published by Karl Pearson in 1899 (Pearson et al. 1899). The issue was later mentioned and made famous in a paper by Edward H. Simpson in 1951, discussing the way in which the relationship between two variables changed after a third variable was factored into a 2 × 2 contingency table (Simpson 1951). When such data are analysed by regression methods, the *reversal paradox* is more often known as *Lord's paradox*, particularly within the behavioural sciences (Lord 1967, 1969), ever since Frederic M. Lord published his paper on this phenomenon with respect to the use of *analysis of covariance* (ANCOVA) in 1967 (Lord 1967). We discussed Lord's paradox in Chapter 4. Within any generalised linear modelling framework, this phenomenon is more generally known in the statistical literature as the *suppression effect*, with the third variable termed a *suppressor* (Horst 1941; Cohen and Cohen 1983; Lewis and Escobar 1986; Lynn 2003; Friedman and Wall 2005).

Thus, in whatever form and under whatever name, the reversal paradox has been recognised ever since the statistical methods of correlation and regression became established. Furthermore, however labelled, this paradox has been extensively explored in the statistical literature, especially within the behavioural sciences (Hand 1994; Lindley 2001), yet, comparatively, none of these analyses acknowledge that they are, in fact, different manifestations of the same phenomenon—that is, they are all just *one* paradox. Moreover, whilst the original definition and naming of the reversal paradox drew on the notion that the direction of any relationship between two variables is reversed after a third variable is introduced, it may nevertheless be generalised to scenarios where the relationship between two such variables is enhanced, *not* reversed *nor* reduced, after a third variable is introduced.

In this chapter the foetal origins of adult disease (FOAD) hypothesis in epidemiology is used to illustrate how the adjustment for a *questionable* confounder on the causal path might give rise to the reversal paradox in linear regression. As this hypothesis will be further used as motivating examples and discussed in later chapters, we give a brief review of the history of the foetal origins hypothesis and its underlying biological theory in this chapter. Then vector geometry is used to illustrate the reversal paradox for this hypothesis. The focus of controversy is whether current body size should be adjusted for when testing the associations between birth size and health outcomes in later life (Huxley et al. 2002).

The statistical adjustment of current body size in the foetal origins hypothesis has been questioned for some time. For instance, Paneth and co-workers (Paneth and Susser 1995; Paneth et al. 1996) specifically addressed the issue of *overcontrolling* for current body mass index when analysing the relation between birth weight and disease risk in later life. In recent years, the results of the adjusted analysis have been given a new meaning; that is, the increased associations between birth size and health outcomes after the adjustment seem to suggest that compensatory, rapid postnatal growth is more important than birth size per se in initiating chronic diseases in later life. This modified theory is called the *developmental origin of health and disease* (DOHaD) *hypothesis*. We will discuss the potential opportunities and challenges in DOHaD hypothesis in Chapters 8 and 9.

7.2 Background: The Foetal Origins of Adult Disease Hypothesis (Barker's Hypothesis)

Inverse associations observed between low birth weight and markers of chronic disease in later life have generated what is termed the *foetal origins of adult disease hypothesis* or *Barker's hypothesis*, so called because it was named after Professor David Barker from the University of Southampton. In the last two decades, numerous epidemiological studies found a reverse relationship between birth weight and the risk of many chronic diseases, such as cardiovascular diseases and hypertension, and this hypothesis became well known within medical and epidemiological communities (Barker and Osmond 1986; Barker 1996). The idea is that an unfavourable environment, or insults (such as poor nutrition) during foetal life, might induce lifetime effects on the subsequent development of bodily systems and hence give rise to major disease processes such as hypertension (Huxley et al. 2000), diabetes (Gluckman and Hanson 2004), asthma (Yuan et al. 2002) and obesity (Leon et al. 1996). The biological theory has been further elaborated in recent years, especially by Professors Peter Gluckman from the University of Auckland, New Zealand, and Mark Hanson from the University of Southampton. These researchers proposed that the biological interaction between foetus and maternal environment via the placenta will have a substantial impact on the later development of chronic diseases. They term this *predictive-adaptive responses* of the foetus (Gluckman and Hanson 2005). For instance, if the foetus receives biological signals, such as high cortisol or insufficient nutrients in the blood, via the placenta from the mother, it might 'predict' that the future environment into which it is to be delivered will match the environment it enjoys at the present time. To survive and adapt to the postnatal environment, the foetus therefore needs to 'choose' the best trajectory of physiological development. However, if the mother provides incorrect biological signals to the foetus via the placenta, or the environment subsequently changes, the trajectory chosen by the foetus might be beneficial to short-term survival in a deprived environment but could potentially put the foetus at a greater risk of suffering various chronic diseases in later life (Gluckman and Hanson 2005). As birth size is the integrated sum of the many foetal experiences, the foetus subjected to many environmental cues suggesting a deprived postnatal environment is more likely to be smaller (Gluckman and Hanson 2005).

Over the last decade, many studies have been undertaken in many parts of the world to examine these proposed relationships (Stein et al. 2005). Although some researchers have questioned the biological basis of the hypothesis as well as its clinical importance (Paneth and Susser 1995), the concept that low birth weight is an independent risk factor for a range of chronic diseases in later life is now widely recognised as scientifically plausible, linked to poor foetal nutrition (Rasmussen 2001). One consequence of this seemingly plausible mechanism is that the foetal origins hypothesis is increasingly viewed as an important issue for public health and preventive medicine (Law 2002).

7.2.1 Epidemiological Evidence on the Foetal Origins Hypothesis

According to the proponents of the hypothesis, numerous epidemiological studies on the foetal origins hypothesis have provided consistent evidence supporting an inverse relation between birth size and adult health outcomes (Barker 2001; Kuh and Ben-Shlomo 2004; Gluckman and Hanson 2005), beginning with ecological studies by Forsdahl (1977) in Norway and by Barker and Osmond (1986) based on data from Hertfordshire in the UK. Historical and cohort studies from Barker's group have replicated these earlier findings (Barker et al. 1989, 1990). An account by Barker can be found in his short article in the *British Medical Journal* (Barker 2003). These associations have also been confirmed by many different groups of investigators in several countries, including the United Kingdom (Frankel et al. 1996, Whincup et al. 1999), the United States (Curhan et al. 1996a, 1996b; Rich-Edward et al. 1997, 1999; Yiu et al. 1999), Sweden (Leon et al. 1998; Carlsson et al. 1999), Finland (Eriksson et al. 1999), India (Fall et al. 1998), Zimbabwe (Woelk et al. 1998), South Africa (Levitt et al. 1999), and Brazil (Barros and Victora 1999).

Although many studies have reported inverse relationships between birth size and health outcomes in later life, these relations have been generally weak and non-substantial (Table 7.1) but become stronger and appear more consistent when current body size is adjusted for in statistical modelling. The practice of adjusting for current body size, however, has caused some controversy (Lucas et al. 1999; Huxley et al. 2002), which we will now go on to discuss by examining the statistical issues behind these practices.

7.2.2 Criticisms of the Foetal Origins Hypothesis

Whilst some early sceptics of FOAD hypothesis were 'converted' by the sheer volume of epidemiological evidence that emerged (Gillman and Rich-Edward 2000), others remained critical of aspects of the statistical techniques that have been used and the way in which studies that support the hypothesis have interpreted their evidence (Paneth and Susser 1995; Paneth et al. 1996; Lucas et al. 1999; Huxley et al. 2002). Two articles outlined substantive challenges faced by the foetal origins hypothesis (Lucas et al. 1999; Huxley et al. 2002). One raised concerns over the statistical methodology used and the improper interpretation of epidemiological analyses invoked in support of the hypothesis (Lucas et al. 1999). The second article suggested that the inverse association between birth weight and adult diseases might 'chiefly reflect the impact of random error' in the measurement of birth weights as well as 'selective emphasis on particular results' (by which they meant publication bias in favour of analyses describing inverse relationships between birth weight (BW) and adult blood pressure (BP)), and 'inappropriate adjustment for current weight and for [other] confounding factors' (Huxley et al. 2002, p. 659). A meta-analysis also indicated that the relationship between blood pressure and birth weight might suffer publication bias because small studies were more likely to report stronger inverse associations (Schluchter 2003). Indeed, whilst a number of retrospective studies have found a direct relationship between birth weight and adult health outcomes, others found that a significant relationship only emerged after adjusting for subsequent body size (notably, current body weight or body mass index) in the statistical analyses.

Current body sizes, such as current body weight (CW), current body height (CH) and current body mass index ($CBMI$), are most frequently adjusted for as alleged confounders in epidemiological studies of the foetal origins hypothesis (Huxley et al. 2002), though little justification for this practice has been provided by these studies. In general, these variables are positively correlated with the outcome measures, such as systolic blood pressure (SBP), and also positively correlated with birth size measures, such as birth weight and birth length. Therefore, proponents of the foetal origins hypothesis argue that these confounders will blur the relation between birth size and adult health outcomes and must therefore be *adjusted for*. However, if current body size is on the causal path from birth size to the health outcomes in later life,

TABLE 7.1

The Reported Correlations between Systolic Blood Pressure (*SBP*) and Body Size Variables and between the Three Body Size Variables in the 37 Studies Included in a Systematic Review by Huxley et al. (2002)

Studies	$r_{BP,BW}$	$r_{BW,CW}$	$r_{BW,CBMI}$	$r_{BW,CH}$	$r_{BP,CW}$	$r_{BP,CH}$	$r_{BP,CBMI}$	$r_{CW,CH}$	$r_{CW,CBMI}$	$r_{CH,CBMI}$	Sex
Law et al. (1993)		0.39 (age = 1); 0.34 (age = 4)									M+F
Law et al. (1993)		0.41	0.12								M+F
Zureik et al. (1996)		0.09		0.1							M+F
Hashimoto et al. (1996)	0.09				0.44						M+F
Levitt et al. (1999)	-0.05				0.22	0.24					M+F
Stocks et al. (1999)	0.06	0.28	0.13	0.32	0.21	0.13	0.16	0.52	0.84	-0.01	M+F
Yiu et al. (1999)	0.03	0.24			0.33	0.2					M+F
Loar et al. (1997)	0.011				0.171	0.081	0.143				M+F
Vancheri et al. (1995)	-0.043	0.323			0.188						M+F
Wincup et al. (1989)	0.003	0.27			0.35						M
Wincup et al. (1989)	0.035										F
Donker et al. (1997)	0.025	0.121		0.087							M+F
Donker et al. (1997)											M+F
Nilsson et al. (1997)		0.21	0.08	0.27							M+F

Source: From Tu Y.K. et al., *Journal of Human Hypertension*, 20, p. 647, 2006. With permission.

Note: BW: birth weight; BP: systolic blood pressure; CW: current body weight; CH: current body height; CBMI: current body mass index; M: males; F: females.

adjustments for it are questionable (see our discussion in Chapter 3). This is because a variable that lies on a causal path from the exposure/risk factor to the outcome is not a *true* confounder (Kirkwood and Sterne 2003; Jewell 2004), even though it might be statistically associated with both the exposure and the outcome variables.

The concept of what constitutes a confounder has been explored extensively in recent years, with greater emphasis given to the definition of *causality* in the associations amongst outcomes, exposures, and confounders (Weinberg 1993). Detailed expositions on this issue have only recently emerged (Pearl 2000; Hernan et al. 2002; Vandenbroucke 2002; Jewell 2004), and these revised definitions of what constitutes a confounder are being increasingly accepted throughout the discipline of epidemiology.

The principal issue of statistical adjustment pertinent to the foetal origins hypothesis is whether or not the adjustment of current body size can help distinguish the effects of birth size on health outcomes via different causal pathways. If one defines a causal path as the chain of events or factors leading in sequence to an outcome, it makes sense to examine an outcome in relation to any one point backward along the *causal* path (McNamee 2003; Jewell 2004). Using the observed inverse relation between birth weight and adult blood pressure as an example, one may differentiate between two different but complementary causal pathways: (1) low birth weight affecting blood pressure *directly* (for instance, poor nutrition or restricted growth in utero having an irreversible impact on the subsequent development of the cardiovascular systems); and (2) low birth weight affecting blood pressure via birth weight's impact on current weight (CW; for instance, through a genetic link between size at birth and current adult body size), which in turn is causally related to high blood pressure (i.e., $BW \rightarrow CW \rightarrow BP$). For the non-converters, it is only sensible to examine *either* the relation between birth weight and adult blood pressure, *or* the relation between current weight and adult blood pressure with the adjustment of BW as a confounder. It is *not* sensible to examine the relation between birth weight and adult blood pressure *whilst controlling for* current weight *as a confounder* since adult weight lies on the causal pathway between the outcome (blood pressure) and the exposure (birth weight). To statistically *adjust* for current weight whilst exploring the impact of birth weight on adult blood pressure invokes the reversal paradox (Stigler 1999). However, for the proponents, the adjustment of current body size reveals two causal effects of birth size on health outcomes: the direct (i.e., $BW \rightarrow BP$) and the indirect (i.e., $BW \rightarrow CW \rightarrow BP$) effect (see Section 3.3 in Chapter 3).

7.2.3 Reversal Paradox and Suppression in Epidemiological Studies on the Foetal Origins Hypothesis

Let us leave aside the debate on whether or not current body size is a genuine confounder for the association between birth size and health outcomes in later life. Instead, we take a look at why results from the unadjusted and adjusted analyses are different from a statistical viewpoint. The standardised regression coefficient in (simple) linear regression is equal to the Pearson product-moment correlation coefficient (r):

$$r = \frac{Cov(x,y)}{\sigma_x \sigma_y},$$ (7.1)

where $Cov(x,y)$ is the covariance of the variables x and y, σ_x is the standard deviation (SD) of x, and σ_y is the SD of y. Let r_{y1} be the bivariate correlation between y and covariate x_1, r_{y2} the bivariate correlation between y and x_2, and r_{12} the bivariate correlation between x_1 and x_2. Within a multiple regression analysis, where y is the dependent variable and x_1 and x_2 are covariates, then $y = b_0 + b_1 x_1 + b_2 x_2 + \varepsilon$. If all variables are standardised by subtracting their means and dividing by the standard deviations of the variables, the standardised partial regression coefficient for x_1 (β_1) is given by

$$\beta_1 = \frac{r_{y1} - r_{12} r_{y2}}{1 - r_{12}^2},$$ (7.2)

and the standardised regression coefficient for x_2 (β_2) is given by

$$\beta_2 = \frac{r_{y2} - r_{12} r_{y1}}{1 - r_{12}^2}.$$ (7.3)

Now suppose that y is the current blood pressure, x_1 is the birth weight, and x_2 is the current weight. For most studies on the foetal origins hypothesis, the bivariate correlation between y and x_1 (r_{y1}) is negative though weak, and for some studies it is occasionally positive though also weak. A few studies do not even bother reporting this bivariate correlation. However, the impact of current weight on health in later life is evident; for example, heavier adults tend to have higher blood pressure, especially systolic pressure. This is perhaps why many studies make a statistical adjustment for current weight when investigating the relation between birth weight and adult blood pressure. Since heavier babies also tend to become heavier in adulthood; that is, there is a positive correlation between birth weight and adult weight (Law et al. 1993; Stokes and Davey Smith 1999), the influence of current weight on blood pressure is considered a confounding factor needing to be 'controlled for' statistically by incorporating current weight within a multiple regression analysis. This is achieved either by incorporating an additional covariate for current weight directly or by incorporating the covariate body mass index. The regression coefficient, β_1, derived after statistical *adjustment* or *control* for current body size, is interpreted as the *independent* contribution of birth weight to current blood pressure (or *direct* effect of birth weight).

From Equation 7.2, it is evident that if r_{y1} is of no significance (i.e., it is very close to zero, irrespective of sign), the numerator will have a good chance of being negative whenever r_{y2} and r_{12} have the same sign because the denominator will always be positive. In this illustration, r_{y2} and r_{12} represent the correlation between current weight and blood pressure and between current weight and birth weight, respectively, and it is almost certain that both are positive. Thus, the magnitude of the negative β_1 depends on r_{y2} and r_{12}. Therefore, the weak negative association between birth weight and blood pressure might be enhanced after adjustment for current body weight, and the weak positive association might be weakened or even reversed.

On other hand, the standardised regression coefficient for current body weight β_2 is very likely to become more positive after adjusting for birth weight. Since r_{y1} is of no significance, β_2 in Equation 6.3 can be reduced to $r_{y2}/(1 - r_{12}^2)$. As $1 - r_{12}^2$ is always smaller than 1, β_2 is, therefore, very likely to be greater than r_{y2}, the bivariate correlation between blood pressure and current body weight. Thus, although birth weight is not strongly correlated with the outcome (blood pressure), incorporating birth weight actually increases the relation between blood pressure and current body weight. The explanation for this phenomenon is that, although birth weight is not strongly correlated with blood pressure, it is positively correlated with current body weight. By adjusting for birth weight, the 'part' of the variation in current body weight that is not correlated with blood pressure is 'suppressed' by birth weight, thereby 'enhancing' the relation between blood pressure and current body weight. This is why, within the statistical literature, suppression is sometimes known as *enhancement* (Lewis and Escobar 1986).

7.2.4 Catch-Up Growth and the Foetal Origins Hypothesis

Inverse associations between birth weight and various chronic adult diseases *after* adjustment of current body sizes have sometimes been interpreted as meaning that *change* in size following birth (i.e., postnatal growth) has a stronger impact on health in later life than birth weight per se. The implication is that babies with lower birth sizes but normal adult body size have greater risk of developing adverse later-life health outcomes (Power et al. 2003).

Change in body size at birth from small to normal (or larger than average) in later life has been termed *catch-up growth* (Ong et al. 2000). However, much of the epidemiological evidence used to support this modified hypothesis is based on similar statistical models as those used to support the foetal origins hypothesis in general; the only difference lies in the interpretation of the statistical model. For instance, considering systolic blood pressure as the adult outcome of interest, most studies only find a significant inverse relationship between blood pressure and birth weight after adjustment for current weight. When adjustment for current body size variables is not made, the relation between birth weight and blood pressure is substantially reduced and is frequently non-significant. For some researchers, this seems to indicate that there is an correlation between birth weight and current body weight, and the corresponding interpretation is that it is more likely to be catch-up growth than birth weight that has an impact on the health outcome since the relation between birth weight and blood pressure is weak without adjustment for current weight (Power et al. 2003). Some studies chose to adjust for change in weight (i.e., weight gain) instead of current body weight (Launer et al. 1993; Stettler et al. 2002). However, the statistical models with birth weight and current body weight, or birth weight and weight change (growth weight), are essentially equivalent (Lucas et al. 1999; see Section 7.3.2), although the partial regression coefficients for birth weight are different. Consider the following model for systolic blood pressure (*SBP*) at age 30 regressed on birth weight (*BW*) and current body weight (*CW*):

$$SBP = b_{10} + b_{11}BW + b_{12}CW + e_1, \qquad \text{(Model 7.1)}$$

where b_{10} is the intercept, b_{11} the regression coefficient for BW, b_{12} the regression coefficient for CW and e_1 the residual error term. If we replace CW with growth in body weight, which is defined as $GW = (CW - BW)$, we obtain the following new model:

$$SBP = b_{20} + b_{21}BW + b_{22}GW + e_2, \qquad \text{(Model 7.2)}$$

where b_{20} is the intercept, b_{21} the regression coefficient for BW, b_{22} the regression coefficient for GW and e_2 the residual error term. If we replace BW with growth in body weight in Model 7.1, we obtain the third model:

$$SBP = b_{30} + b_{31}GW + b_{32}CW + e_3, \qquad \text{(Model 7.3)}$$

where b_{30} is the intercept, b_{31} is the regression coefficient for GW, b_{32} is the regression coefficient for CW and e_3 is the residual error term. In fact, as shown by Lucas et al. (1999) and other studies (Keijzer-Veen et al. 2005; Tu et al. 2006a), these three models are mathematically related. For instance, by substituting CW with $(BW + GW)$, Model 7.1 can be rearranged as

$$SBP = b_{10} + b_{11}BW + b_{12}(BW + GW) + e_1$$

$$SBP = b_{10} + (b_{11} + b_{12})BW + b_{12}GW + e_1$$

As a result, b_{21} in Model 7.2 is the sum of b_{11} and b_{12}, and b_{22} is equal to b_{12}. By substituting BW with $(CW - GW)$, Model 7.1 can be rearranged as

$$SBP = b_{10} + b_{11}(CW - GW) + b_{12}CW + e_1$$

$$SBP = b_{10} + 9 - b_{11})GW + (b_{11} + b_{12})CW + e_1$$

As a result, b_{31} in Model 7.3 is $-b_{11}$, and b_{32} is the sum of b_{11} and b_{12}. These three models have the same R^2 and three residual errors term (Tu et al. 2006a). The key question is how the results from these models should be interpreted. For instance, the regression coefficient for *BW* is b_{11} in Model 7.1 but $(b_{11} + b_{12})$ in Model 7.2; which is the *real* effect of *BW* on *SBP*?

Due to the potential problems with the interpretation of multiple regression models, Cole (2004) used his lifecourse plot to argue that, as the effect of body weight on the health outcome, such as systolic blood pressure, changes from a small inverse effect to a stronger positive effect, the change in weight has a stronger influence on adult health than early weight (Adair and Cole 2005; Cole 2005). We will discuss the lifecourse plot and other more complex approaches in Chapters 9 and 10.

Instead of modelling weight change in kilograms, some studies use changes in z-scores of body weights (Ley et al. 1997), such as the difference between birth weight z-scores and current weight z-scores, and this was considered an index of catch-up growth. Therefore, if babies with a negative z-score for birth weight grow to adulthood with a positive z-score for current body weight, they have a positive change in z-score body weight, indicating catch-up growth.

Nevertheless, the variance of birth weight in kilograms is far smaller than that of current weight in kilograms, with variations in weight at birth within a few kilograms, increasing with age. Thus, those with low birthweight z-scores and only slightly increased current-weight z-scores might in fact gain less weight (in kilograms) than those with high birth-weight z-scores and only slightly decreased current-weight z-scores. Consequently, the relation between blood pressure and growth weight in kilograms might be different from that between blood pressure and growth weight expressed in terms of z-scores. It is less clear how to interpret the impact of changes in z-scores, as opposed to changes in kilograms, upon the function of the human body. From a statistical viewpoint, the relation between blood pressure and change in body weight can be expressed as

$$r_{y,z-x} = \frac{r_{yz}s_z - r_{yx}s_x}{\sqrt{(s_x^2 + s_z^2 - 2r_{xz}s_xs_z)}},$$

(7.4)

where y is blood pressure, x is birth weight, z is current body weight, r_{yx} is the correlation between blood pressure and birth weight, r_{yz} is the correlation between blood pressure and current body weight, r_{xz} the correlation between birth weight and current body weight, s_x is the standard deviation of birth weight, s_y is the standard deviation of blood pressure, and s_z is the standard deviation of current body weight. As the correlation between blood pressure and birth weight (r_{yx}) is often weak, Equation 7.4 can be simplified as

$$r_{y,z-x} \approx \frac{r_{yz}s_z}{\sqrt{(s_x^2 + s_z^2 - 2r_{xz}s_xs_z)}} . \tag{7.5}$$

Therefore, the correlation between blood pressure and change in body weight (i.e., weight gain after birth, or growth weight) is dominated by the correlation between blood pressure and current body weight. If changes in z-scores of body weights are used instead of changes in actual body weights in kilograms, Equation 7.5 can be further simplified as

$$r_{y,z-x} \approx \frac{r_{yz}}{\sqrt{2(1-r_{xz})}} . \tag{7.6}$$

It is noted that when the correlation between birth weight and current body weight (r_{xz}) is greater than 0.5, $r_{y,z-x}$ will be greater than r_{yz}; that is, were there no relation between birth weight and blood pressure, using change in (z-score) weights derived by subtracting (z-score) birth weight from (z-score) current body weight might yield a strong association with blood pressure.

7.2.5 Residual Current Body Weight: A Proposed Alternative Approach

Recently, an alternative regression model has been proposed to overcome the problem of adjustment for current body weight (Keijzer-Veen et al. 2005). Instead of adjusting for current body weight, the unexplained residual current body weight (CW_{res}) should be adjusted for, where CW_{res} is the set of residuals of the simple regression model where current body weight is regressed on birth weight. Keijzer-Veen et al. (2005) considered CW_{res} to be the unexplained (by birth weight) current body weight. They recognised that the adjustment for current body weight might not be justified at all since it is on the causal path, and they preferred this approach because it estimates the effects of birth weight and the effect of additional weight gain in a single model.

Algebraically, as CW_{res} is the set of residuals for current body weight regressed on birth weight, the correlation between CW_{res} and birth weight should be zero. When blood pressure is regressed on birth weight and CW_{res}, from Equation 7.2, $\beta_{BP.BW|CWres}$, the standardised partial regression coefficient for birth weight is given by

$$\beta_{BP.BW|CWres} = \frac{r_{RP,BW} - r_{BW,CWres}r_{BP,CWres}}{1 - r_{BW,CWres}^2} , \tag{7.7}$$

where $r_{BP,BW}$ is the correlation between blood pressure and birth weight; $r_{BP,CWres}$ is the correlation between blood pressure and CW_{res}; and $r_{BW,CWres}$ is the correlation between birth weight and CW_{res}. As $r_{BW,CWres}$ is zero, $\beta_{BP.BW|CWres}$ is equivalent to $r_{BP,BW}$, and the partial regression coefficient for birth weight, $b_{BP.BW|CWres}$ ($= \beta_{BP.BW|CWres}*(s_{BP}/s_{BW})$), where s_{BP} is the standard deviation of blood pressure and s_{BW} the standard deviation of birth weight) is equivalent to the simple regression coefficient for birth weight when blood pressure is regressed on birth weight. It is noted that the P-value for $\beta_{BP.BW|CWres}$ is larger than $r_{BP,BW}$ due to loss of one degree of freedom in the multiple regression. Furthermore, the partial regression coefficient for CW_{res}, $b_{BP.CWres|BW}$, is equivalent to the simple regression coefficient for CW_{res}, $b_{BP.CWres}$, when blood pressure is regressed on CW_{res}, and also equivalent to the partial regression coefficient for current weight, $b_{BP.CW|BW}$, when blood pressure is regressed on birth weight and current weight.

In other words, from our discussions thus far, it is clear that the proposed model is just a rearrangement of commonly used statistical models (Lucas et al. 1999; Tu et al. 2006a) in the foetal origins hypothesis. This approach therefore fails to overcome the problem of adjustment for current body weight, as originally intended (Keijzer-Veen et al. 2005).

7.2.6 Numerical Example

We use the statistical package R to simulate data for a hypothetical sample of 100 adult males based on information in the literature (Hennessey and Alberman 1998) and surveys conducted by the UK Department of Health in 2002 (http://www.doh.gov.uk). Simulated variables are birth weight (*BW*), with mean = 3.5 kg and standard deviation (SD) = 0.6 kg; blood pressure (*BP*), with mean = 129.4 mmHg, SD = 11.7 mmHg; and current weight (*CW*), with mean = 81.2 kg, SD = 14.3 kg. Data are simulated such that the correlation between birth weight and blood pressure is negative but very close to zero ($r_{BW-BP} = -0.008$), the correlation between birth and current weights is modestly positive ($r_{BW-CW} = 0.160$), and current weight and blood pressure are substantially correlated ($r_{CW-BP} = 0.500$).

Blood pressure regressed on birth weight only confirms that there is no evidence of an association (Table 7.2): regression coefficient for *BW* = –0.156 mmHg/kg [95% confidence interval (CI) = –4.055, 3.743; P = 0.937]. Blood pressure regressed on current weight only confirms a relationship (Table 7.2): regression coefficient for *CW* = 0.413 mmHg/kg [95% CI = 0.272, 0.555; P < 0.001]. Now, following the practice of many previous studies, blood pressure is regressed on birth weight and current weight simultaneously (Table 7.2, Model 7.1): regression coefficients for *BW* = –1.775 mmHg/kg [95% CI = –5.18, 1.631; P = 0.304] and for *CW* = 0.425 mmHg/kg [95% CI = 0.282, 0.568; P < 0.001]. Following adjustment for current weight, the inverse association between blood pressure and birth weight increases. Not only does the negative effect of birth weight on blood pressure increase from 0.156 to 1.775 mmHg/kg but the positive impact of current weight also increases from 0.413 to 0.425 mmHg/kg.

TABLE 7.2

Simple and Multiple Regression Models for Simulated Hypothetical Data on Birth Weight, Blood Pressure, and Current Body Weight

		Regression Coefficients (95% CI)	P-value	R^2
	Intercept	129.9	—[a]	<0.001
	Birth weight (BW)	−0.156 (−4.055, 3.743)	0.937	
	Intercept	95.8	—[a]	0.256
	Current weight (CW)	0.413 (0.272, 0.555)	<0.001	
Model 7.1	Intercept	101.1	—[a]	0.264
	Birth weight (BW)	−1.775 (−5.18, 1.631)	0.304	
	Current weight (CW)	0.425 (0.282, 0.568)	<0.001	
Model 7.2	Intercept	101.1	—[a]	0.264
	Birth weight (BW)	−1.349 (−4.735, 2.036)	0.431	
	Growth weight (GW)	0.425 (0.282, 0.568)	<0.001	
Model 7.3	Intercept	101.1	—[a]	0.264
	Growth weight (GW)	1.775 (−4.735, 2.036)	0.304	
	Current weight (CW)	−1.349 (−1.631, 5.180)	0.431	

Note: The dependent variable in all models is *BP*.

[a] It is trivial to test the significance of the intercept.

Alternatively, we regress blood pressure (*BP*) on birth weight (*BW*) and growth weight (*GW*) (Table 7.2, Model 7.2): regression coefficients for *BW* = −1.349 mmHg/kg [95% CI = −4.735, 2.036; *P* = 0.431] and for *GW* = 0.425 mmHg/kg [95% CI = 0.282, 0.568; *P* < 0.001]; or we regress blood pressure (*BP*) on growth weight (*GW*) and current weight (*CW* Table 7.2, Model 7.3): regression coefficients for *GW* = 1.775 mmHg/kg [95% CI = −4.735, 2.036; *P*=0.304] and for *CW* = −1.349 [95% CI = −1.631, 5.180; *P* = 0.431]. Regression coefficient absolute values, associated 95% CIs, *P*-values, and model fit (assessed by R^2) are identical for birth weight (Model 7.1) and growth weight (Model 7.3), identical for current weight (Model 7.1) and growth weight (Model 7.2), and identical for birth weight (Model 7.2) and current weight (Model 7.3).

7.3 Vector Geometry of the Foetal Origins Hypothesis

In this section we use vector geometry to illustrate the reversal paradox in the foetal origins hypothesis and associated interpretations. We use adult systolic blood pressure (*SBP*) as the outcome, with birth weight (*BW*) and adult current weight (*CW*) as potential covariates. For simplicity, all four variables are treated as continuous. An additional covariate of catch-up growth/

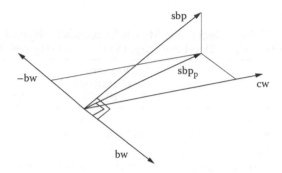

FIGURE 7.1
Vector illustration of multiple regression for blood pressure, regressed simultaneously on birth weight and current weight. If **sbp** is orthogonal to **bw**, the projection of **sbp** to the subspace spanned by **bw** and **cw** (**sbp**$_p$) will also be orthogonal to **bw**.

growth weight (*GW*) is defined as the difference between current weight and birth weight (*CW* – *BW*).

In this section we also use vector geometry to illustrate the relationships amongst blood pressure (*SBP*), birth weight (*BW*), and current weight (*CW*) in Model 7.1. In geometry, we consider the vectors, **sbp**, **bw** and **cw**, respectively, where the correlation between blood pressure and birth weight is nearly zero ($r_{SBP,BW} \approx 0$); hence, **sbp** and **bw** are almost orthogonal. If **sbp** and **bw** are orthogonal, the projection of *sbp* (**sbp**$_p$) on the plane spanned by **bw** and **cw** is also orthogonal to **bw** (Figure 7.1). Within the multiple regression model **sbp**$_p = b_{BW}$**bw** + b_{CW}**cw**, the partial regression coefficient for birth weight (b_{BW}) is derived using the parallelogram rule by projecting **sbp**$_p$ onto the vector **bw** parallel to the direction of **cw** (Figure 7.1). Consequently, b_{BW} is not zero but negative due to the positive angle between both **sbp** and **cw** and between **bw** and **cw**. In terms of variables, b_{BW} is negative due to the positive correlations between blood pressure and birth weight, and between current weight and birth weight.

In general, the smaller the angle between **bp** and **cw** (i.e., the greater the positive correlation between blood pressure and current weight) and/or the smaller the angle between **bw** and **cw** (i.e., the greater the positive correlation between birth weight and current weight), the greater the length of the projection of **sbp**$_p$ on **bw** along the vector **cw** (i.e., the greater the absolute value of b_{BW}). Furthermore, although the partial regression coefficient for birth weight (b_{BW}) is not zero when blood pressure is regressed simultaneously on birth weight and current weight, the former nevertheless contributes nothing to 'explain' the variance in blood pressure. This is because birth weight and blood pressure are uncorrelated (orthogonal in vector space). The proportion of variance in *BP* explained by *BW* and *CW* (measured by R^2, which is equal to ($\|$**sbp**$_p\|/\|$**bp**$\|^2$) is given as (Bring 1996)

$$R^2 = r_{y1} * \beta_1 + r_{y2} * \beta_2 , \tag{7.8}$$

where β_1 and β_2 are the standardised regression coefficients for BW and CW (see Equations 7.2 and 7.3), and r_{y1} and r_{y2} are the correlations between BP and BW and between BP and CW, respectively. As r_{y1} is nearly zero, though b_{BW} (therefore, β_1) is not zero, BW contributes nothing to the explained variance of SBP. Readers can find the vector geometry for Models 7.2 and 7.3 in our previous study (Tu et al. 2006a).

7.4 Reversal Paradox and Adjustment for Current Body Size: Empirical Evidence from Meta-Analysis

In Sections 7.2 and 7.3 we discuss the controversy of the reversal paradox in the foetal origin hypothesis from a statistical and geometrical perspective. Our discussion indicates that the reversal paradox may be a serious problem in the interpretation of the association between birth size and health outcomes in later life. We have also undertaken simulation studies to illustrate the potential impact of the reversal paradox (Tu et al. 2005d; Tu et al. 2006b), and the results from our simulations are consistent with our theoretical expositions. We have also undertaken a meta-analysis to investigate the extent of this problem in epidemiological research (Tu et al. 2006b).

In our meta-analysis, we examined the 37 studies included in a previous systematic review (Huxley et al. 2002) to identify any that had reported regression coefficients for birth weight (BW) when systolic blood pressure (SBP) in later life was regressed on BW before and/or after adjustment for one or more measures of current body size. For each statistical model reported, data were collected on any adjustments made for one or more measures of current body size and on the reported effect sizes (i.e., partial regression coefficients of BW) when SBP was regressed on BW. Weighted estimates were then combined using the statistical software package Stata (Stata Corporation, College Station, Texas) to perform both fixed- and random-effect meta-analyses because there is no consensus on whether the fixed-effects model or the random-effects model is better (Egger et al. 2001). A previous meta-analysis reported substantial heterogeneity amongst these studies (Huxley et al. 2002), and we therefore chose to explore findings from either approach.

In studies reporting an unadjusted *negative* association between BW and BP, the association was strengthened after adjusting for current body size. Similarly, amongst studies reporting an unadjusted *positive* association between BW and BP, the association was either diminished or reversed (i.e., the association between BW and BP became negative) after adjusting for current body size. In both instances, the impact of adjusting for one measure of current body size was enhanced following adjustments for additional measures of current body size. One study (Stocks and Davey Smith 1999) adjusted for three measures of current body size (*CW, CH* and *CBMI*) and observed that the positive unadjusted relationship between *BW* and *BP* was initially diminished and then became negative, but only after adjusting for successive measures of current body size.

Within a fixed-effects meta-analysis, the pooled estimate of changes in systolic blood pressure per 1 kg increase in birth weight was, without adjustment for any measures of current body size, −0.64 mmHg/kg (95% CI = −0.74, −0.54). Within a random-effects meta-analysis this was −0.31 mmHg/kg (95% CI = −0.82, 0.20). Generally, pooled estimates moved away from zero following adjustment for just one measure of current body size. The fixed-effects estimate was −0.72 mmHg/kg (95% CI = −0.77, −0.68) and the random-effects estimate was −1.32 mmHg/kg (95% CI = −1.62, −1.03). After adjusting for two measures of current body size, the pooled estimates moved farther from zero: the fixed-effects estimate became −1.53 mmHg/kg (95% CI = −1.20, −1.86) and the random-effects estimate became −1.62 mmHg/kg (95% CI = −2.17, −1.07).

There was substantial heterogeneity within each of three groups (I2 = 81.4%, 94.2% and 55.0%; Q = 86.1, 572.6 and 24.4; $P < 0.001$, $P < 0.001$ and $P = 0.011$; without adjustment for any measure of current body size, adjustment for one measure, and adjustment for two measures, respectively). Egger et al. (2001) tests showed that there was no statistically significant small-study bias for groups either without adjustment for any measure of current body size ($P = 0.321$) or with adjustment for two measures ($P = 0.339$), but Egger et al. (2001) test showed there was a significant small-study bias for the group with adjustment for one measure ($P = 0.028$). The greatest difference in the pooled estimates of the impact of birth weight on blood pressure between the fixed- and random-effects meta-analyses was found in those studies where one current body size was adjusted for.

7.5 Discussion

7.5.1 The Reversal Paradox and the Foetal Origins Hypothesis

In the foetal origins hypothesis literature, body size measurements (be they body weight, body height, or BMI) are frequently considered to be confounders for health-related outcomes. However, there appears to be no consistent practice within the literature as to when and how such variables should (or should not) be 'controlled for', and most studies do not offer any justification for their choice of confounders.

Potentially, the reversal paradox invokes bias due to the inappropriate 'controlling' of alleged confounders that are not, in fact, true confounders (Hernan et al. 2002; Kirkwood and Sterne 2003; Jewell 2004). Whether or not the reversal paradox caused by adjusting for current body size is a problem in the foetal origins hypothesis depends upon the underlying causal models adopted (Arah 2008). For instance, Weinberg proposed a more complex causal model for the foetal origins hypothesis (Weinberg 2005), and under some assumptions, the adjustment for current body weight might be justified for testing the relation between birth weight and blood pressure. However, Weinberg's causal model is one of many possible causal models linking prenatal factors, birth weight, current weight, and blood pressure (Arah 2008; Tu et al. 2008b). Whilst some causal models seem more plausible than others, it is crucial to acknowledge that several feasible models exist. For many proponents of the FOAD hypothesis, current weight is seen as a confounder because there is at least a possibility (in one or more potential causal models) that adjustment for current weight is justified. However, until we have clearer evidence from experimental studies (Ceesay et al. 1997), and a greater understanding of the complex anatomical, physiological and biochemical processes linking birth weight, current weight, and blood pressure (Gluckman and Hanson 2004), all causal models will remain subject to debate. Epidemiological studies need to be more transparent and rigorous in their reports of the formulation of their research questions, the underlining biological mechanisms assumed and the statistical testing adopted of specific research hypotheses stated *a priori* (Lucas et al. 1999; Huxley et al. 2002).

Although birth weight itself is just a proxy variable for foetal growth, it is not always clear in the foetal origins hypothesis what birth weight is a proxy for. The most commonly given interpretation for the linear (i.e., across the whole range of birth weight) inverse relation between birth weight and adult health outcomes is that restricted foetal growth due to 'sub-optimal' nutrition constrains the development of vital organ systems in the foetus and triggers chronic diseases in later life (Gluckman and Hanson 2005). According to Gluckman and Hanson (2005), this is the predictive-adaptive response of the foetus to its maternal environment by *choosing* a different trajectory of physiological development in order to have a better chance of survival in a deprived postnatal environment. Often the result of this predictive-adaptive response is a reduced birth size, which is associated with a reduced adult size. This is a seemingly simple but in fact hardly a refutable concept. A key feature of the foetal origins hypothesis is that no threshold criterion (such as 2.5 kg) is given to define low birth weight, and therefore, any baby can be a relatively low birth weight baby compared to extremely large babies. Thus, low birth weight is a relative concept, and the restricted growth in the uterus measured by birth size also becomes a relative concept. To explain the linear relation between birth size and health hazards in later life, some proponents of the foetal origins hypothesis argue that babies with birthweight of 4.0 kg might have suffered restricted growth if they should have been born with a birthweight of 4.2 kg, just like babies who were born with a birthweight of 2.8 kg but should have been born with a birthweight of 3.0 kg (Gluckman and Hanson 2005). They argue that the difference is that more babies born with 2.8 kg are growth restricted (Gluckman and Hanson 2005). The vital problem is that this argument/theory refers to individual prenatal growth potential/ trajectory, and it is hardly possible (indeed probably impossible) to scientifi- cally refute or prove this counterfactual argument because it is impossible to measure whether or not a baby achieves his or her optimal growth in the uterus; it is impossible to ascertain what is the appropriate nutrition for optimal growth in the uterus. What experiments or statistical analysis show are the average effects of any intervention or exposure. Furthermore, it is still questionable that the linear inverse relation between birth weight and adult disease outcomes observed in epidemiological studies could be interpreted in this way.

Take blood pressure in our simulated example. Notwithstanding adjust- ment for current body weight being questionable, the reverse relation between birth weight and blood pressure in the regression analysis indicated that blood pressure in later life could be reduced by increasing birth weight. The linear reverse relation does not suggest that an individual baby needs optimal nutrition to achieve his or her full growth potential. Instead, this linear inverse relation suggests that the bigger the baby, the lower the risk of chronic diseases in later life. Obviously, it is naïve to suggest that the bigger the baby, the better because the very largest babies run the risk of greater perinatal mortality (Wilcox 2001). Furthermore, some epidemiological stud- ies show that there is a positive relation between birth weight (Hjalgrim et al. 2003) and the risks of both childhood leukaemia and breast cancer in adult women (Michels et al. 1996). The argument/theory purported by the foetal origins hypothesis can only gain credence from experimental intervention studies that have been conducted in animals (Gluckman and Hanson 2005; McMillen and Robinson 2005). For ethical reasons, interventions that can be tested in humans are limited; for example, some studies have compared the health outcomes and cognitive development in babies who were given for- mula milk or who were breastfed (Lucas et al. 1998; Singhal et al. 2001, 2007).

It is worth noting that the estimated effect size in our simulated study, or in any empirical study, is affected by the sample ratio of the blood pressure SD to that of the birth weight SD. If this ratio is large in any particular study, for instance, where the adult age range is wide and thereby yields a wider range of adult blood pressures, the effect size (i.e., the extent of bias) caused by the reversal paradox will be exaggerated. On the other hand, if the sample ratio of blood pressure SD to birth weight SD is small, as, for instance amongst studies of children or young adults, where blood pressure variation tends to be smaller than amongst older adults, the effect size caused by the rever- sal paradox will be diminished. Nevertheless, testing the significance of an association is affected by sample size, and it is well known that even a small effect size will be statistically significant if the sample size is large enough. Most studies examining the foetal origins of adult blood pressure have suf- ficiently large samples to yield statistical significance for relatively small effect sizes. Thus, the exaggerating effect of the reversal paradox tends to give the misleading impression that the relationship between blood pressure and birth weight, after adjustment for current weight, is not only statistically significant (due to the power available to detect the biased difference from zero) but also biologically and clinically significant (as a result of the biased effect size caused or enhanced by the reversal paradox).

7.5.2 Multiple Adjustments for Current Body Sizes

Our meta-analyses provided empirical evidence that the adjustment for current body size when exploring the relationship between birth weight and blood pressure tends to reverse any positive bivariate correlation and strengthen any negative bivariate correlation between these two variables. Unfortunately, not all the studies reported regression coefficients for birth weight when blood pressure was regressed on birth weight both before *and* after adjusting for one or more measures of current body size. Indeed, three of the larger studies only reported effect sizes *after* adjusting for current BMI (Curhan et al. 1996a, 1996b; Nilsson et al. 1997). However, studies that did provide these statistics found that adjustment for successive measures of current body size consistently enhanced pre-existing negative associations between birth weight and blood pressure, and weakened or reversed pre-existing positive associations between birth weight and blood pressure.

Few studies justified their adjustment for one or more measures of current body size. The majority of studies adjusted for just one measure of current body size (most often BMI or body weight) though a smaller number adjusted for both current body weight and current body height, or current body mass index and current body height. A more recent study (Kumar et al. 2004) has since reported regression models before and after adjusting for current BMI, body height and body weight with effect sizes of birth weight and blood pressure increasing from -0.665 mmHg/kg (pre-adjustment) through -0.898 mmHg/kg (after adjusting for current BMI), and -1.705 mmHg/kg (after adjusting for current BMI and body height) to -1.871 mmHg/kg (after adjusting for current BMI, body height and body weight)—very much as our simulations and meta-analyses predict. It is thus difficult, if not impossible, to compare results across studies where so many varied attempts have been made to control for confounders without consistent reasoning concerning the choice of these confounders. This does not invalidate the foetal origins hypothesis per se; rather, it implies that any direct interpretation of inverse relationships between birth weight and *any* adult condition, whilst adjusting for current adult body measurements, cannot be taken to mean that birth weight has a direct impact on the adult outcome.

It is not clear why this more recent study, or a number of the earlier studies, adjusted for more than one measure of current body size. It might be that the negative association expected between birth weight and blood pressure was only evident (or became enhanced and statistically significant) after adjusting for more than one measure of current body size. The latter seems likely for at least some of the studies examined, given that Huxley et al. (2002) found that smaller studies were more likely to report a negative relationship between birth weight and blood pressure—a trend they took to be evidence of publication bias—and our meta-analyses confirm that smaller studies tended to report a more negative relationship between birth weight and blood pressure irrespective of how many measures of current body size measures they adjusted for.

7.5.3 Catch-Up Growth and the Foetal Origins Hypothesis

Lucas et al. (1999) discussed some of the algebraic relationships of regression coefficients amongst the three multivariable models (Models 7.1, 7.2 and 7.3). In this chapter, vector geometry was used to reveal that these three models are effectively equivalent; not only do partial regression coefficients exhibit algebraic relationships but also coefficient *P*-values and model fit (i.e., the explained variance in the outcome, blood pressure) are identical. The crucial issue, therefore, remains with the interpretation of these models. For instance, when birth weight is adjusted for, it is impossible to differentiate the effects of growth weight from that of current weight on blood pressure, since using either covariate gives rise to identical coefficients, *P*-values and explained variance in blood pressure. Conversely, following adjustment for current weight, the impact of growth weight on blood pressure is identical to that of birth weight, albeit in the opposite direction. Thus, the 'independent' impact of growth weight on blood pressure is open to interpretation.

From a clinical viewpoint, adjusting for birth weight (i.e., holding birth weight constant), greater weight gain during life corresponds to greater current weight. Therefore, to argue that weight gain has any impact on blood pressure is equivalent to arguing that current weight has an impact, which, of course, it does. Adjusting for current weight will create a stronger inverse relation between birth weight and blood pressure, though, at the same time, the positive relation between blood pressure and current weight will become stronger. Therefore, it might be growth weight that contributes to elevated blood pressure, though it could also be current weight that affects blood pressure, or both. The apparently stronger effect of current weight on blood pressure after adjustment for birth weight might be interpreted as either the impact of weight is accumulative and linear (which is what the modified hypothesis implies), or that most people with greater body size were also born bigger and, therefore, by removing the *protective* effect of their birth weight, the impact of current weight becomes greater. In contrast, holding current weight constant, those with greater weight gain must have a lower birth weight; hence, the greater the catch-up growth, the higher the adult blood pressure is. As we see from the comparison of Models 7.1 to 7.3, growth weight can be a proxy for either current weight (by adjusting for birth weight) or birth weight (by adjusting for current weight). Consequently, the role of growth weight in the regression models commonly adopted for the foetal origins hypothesis is ambiguous.

However, for the relation between birth weight and blood pressure, whether to adjust for growth weight or current body weight will give rise to different regression coefficients for birth weight. In general, adjusting for growth weight will yield a weaker negative relation between birth weight and blood pressure. Therefore, the question remains: should we adjust for current body weight or growth weight?

7.6 Conclusion

As an understated and poorly recognised issue, the reversal paradox, in whatever form it takes, has the potential to impact severely on data analyses undertaken within empirical research, which increasingly rely upon the methods of generalised linear modelling of observational (i.e., non-randomised) data. It should be noted that the aim of this chapter is not to refute the foetal origins hypothesis, as it may be argued that the version of this hypothesis discussed in this chapter is merely oversimplified. Our discussion should not be seen as criticism of the foetal origins hypothesis but a reminder to epidemiologists that, to arrive at the correct interpretation of evidence supporting or refuting this hypothesis, one must fully understand the statistical methods employed and the implications of making any statistical adjustment for confounders. In Chapter 8, we will discuss specific models proposed for testing the foetal origins hypothesis, and in Chapter 9 we will discuss recent attempts at developing and modifying the foetal origins hypothesis.

8

Testing Statistical Interaction

8.1 Introduction: Testing Interactions in Epidemiological Research

According to one textbook, the definition of *interaction* in epidemiology is 'to describe a situation in which two or more risk factors modify the effect of each other with regard to the occurrence or level of a given outcome' (Szklo and Nieto 2004). This phenomenon is also known as *effect modification* (Szklo and Nieto 2004), as the effect of one risk factor on the health outcome is different across the levels of another risk factor, where the latter is often called an effect modifier of the former. To test statistically whether or not there is interaction between two risk factors, the most frequently used method is to incorporate a product term of the two risk factors; that is, multiplying the exposure variable by the effect modifier variable, in a regression model (Selvin 1994; Kirkwood and Sterne 2003; Szklo and Nieto 2004). If the regression coefficient for the product term is significantly different from zero, this indicates that the effect of one exposure is dependent upon (i.e., modified by) the levels of the effect modifier. Another approach is to stratify the effect modifier and to compare the effect sizes of the exposure variables across a different stratum of the effect modifier (Rothman 2002). These two approaches are equivalent mathematically if the effect modifier is a categorical variable. When the effect modifier is a continuous variable, a common practice is to categorise it into two or more groups and then to test whether or not the effect sizes are different across these groups.

In cancer epidemiology, the testing of interaction is a common statistical practice to explore whether there is any synergistic or antagonistic effect between several exposures. For example, the main risk factors for oral cancer, such as squamous cell carcinoma, are alcohol drinking and cigarette smoking in Western countries, but in some South Asian countries, chewing betel nuts is associated with a high risk of oral cancers. In Taiwan, the habit of chewing betel nuts is popular with people from lower socio-economic backgrounds and they are also more likely to be smokers and drinkers (Wen et al.

2010). The combination of these risk factors may have a synergistic effect in causing oral cancer. In genetic epidemiology, many researchers look for the interaction between genetic markers and environmental exposures; that is, where the risk of developing certain diseases may be greater amongst people with one or more specific genetic polymorphisms under the same conditions of environmental exposure.

Although testing the interaction between explanatory variables is straightforward to implement by incorporating the product terms within statistical models, the interpretation and biological explanation of interaction effects are sometimes challenging. First, there are technical problems, such as measurement errors in the observed variables, which may dilute or change the effects of the interaction. Second, it is less straightforward to determine the meaningful effect size for interactions and to calculate the required sample size for revealing the interaction. Third, and more fundamentally, the testing of statistical interaction is rarely equivalent to testing biological interaction. From a statistical viewpoint, the concept of effect modification (synergistic or antagonistic) is quite clear for a binary outcome (i.e., with or without disease), as it simply means that the difference in odds for people to develop disease with a history of different levels of exposure is related to the levels experienced of the effect modifiers. Using oral cancer as an example, suppose that the odds ratio amongst smokers (versus non-smokers) is 3; if there is no interaction between smoking and betel nut chewing, the odds ratio for smokers versus non-smokers in betel nut users is the same as that in betel nut non-users, and both is 3. However, if there is an interaction, we may find that the odds ratio for smokers versus non-smokers in betel nut users is 8, whilst the odds ratio amongst smokers in betel nut non-users is only 2.5. However, suppose we do not know the carcinogenic mechanism of smoking or betel nut chewing in the pathogenesis of oral cancer. How often can the statistical testing of the product term be interpreted as the evidence of a biological interaction between the smoking of cigarettes and the chewing of betel nuts?

The aim of this chapter is to explain the general concept of testing statistical interaction and demonstrate a little-known statistical concept regarding the testing of a product interaction term between two continuous explanatory variables in a linear regression model when the outcome is also continuous. When these three variables are multivariate normally distributed, the expected value of the partial regression coefficient for the product interaction (between the two covariates) is zero. Then we discuss results from simulations showing the consequence of categorizing the originally continuous exposure and/or effect modifier variables when testing their interaction. Again, we use the foetal origins hypothesis (see Chapter 7) to illustrate the importance of testing statistical interaction in epidemiological research.

8.1 Testing Statistical Interaction between Categorical Variables

We first use a hypothetical example to illustrate how to interpret results from testing statistical interaction between two categorical variables. Table 8.1 shows the associations between the prevalence of oral cancer and the two risk factors (smoking and using betel nut) in a hypothetical cross-sectional survey. The odds ratio of oral cancers for smoking (smokers versus non-smokers) is 3.84 (95% confidence intervals [CI] = 3.20, 4.61), and the odds ratio for using betel nut (yes versus no) is 4.32 (95% CI: 3.60, 5.20). When a multi-variable logistic regression is carried out, the results are given as

$$\text{logit}(\pi) = -5.83 + 0.718\,\text{smoking} + 0.975\,\text{betel nut}, \qquad (8.1)$$

where π is the risk for oral cancer; for example, the prevalence rate. The logit is the log of the prevalence over one minus the prevalence; that is, the *log odds* of having the disease. Equation 8.1 shows that the log odds of oral cancer is a linear function of smoking and betel nut chewing. For people neither smoking nor chewing betel nut, the estimated odds of having oral cancer is the exponential of $(-5.83) = 0.003$. The odds ratio for smoking; that is, the multiplier by which the odds of having oral cancer is increased amongst smokers, is the exponential of $(0.718) = 2.05$ (95% CI = 1.58, 2.66), and the odds ratio for using betel nut is the exponential of $(0.975) = 2.65$ (95% CI = 2.04, 3.44), suggesting that both are independent risk factors for oral cancer. However, the logistic regression model in Equation 8.1 assumes that the elevated odds of having oral cancer due to using betel nut are the same for smokers and non-smokers, and the elevated odds of oral cancer due to smoking are the same for users and non-users of betel nut. For example, according to Equation 8.1,

TABLE 8.1

Prevalence of Oral Cancer in a Hypothetical Population

Oral Cancer	Smoking	Betel Nut Chewing	Number of People
Yes	1	1	150
Yes	1	0	30
Yes	0	1	25
Yes	0	0	300
No	1	1	9,000
No	1	0	6,000
No	0	1	4,000
No	0	0	100,000

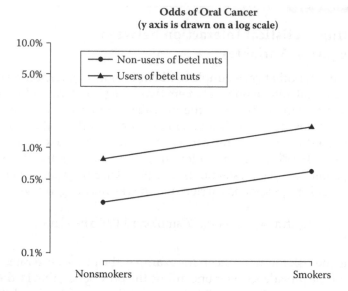

FIGURE 8.1
The relation between the odds of oral cancer and using betel nut in smokers and non-smokers estimated by logistic regression.

the odds of having oral cancer amongst smokers who do not use betel nut is exp(−5.83 + 0.718) = 0.006, and the odds of having oral cancer amongst smokers who use betel nut are exp(−5.83 + 0.718 + 0.975) = 0.016. The odds of oral cancer amongst non-smokers who do not use betel nut are exp(−5.83) = 0.003, and the odds amongst non-smokers who use betel nut are exp(−5.83 + 0.975) = 0.0078. Figure 8.1 shows the estimated relationship between the odds of oral cancer and smoking stratified by betel nut use. In the figure, the vertical axis for odds is on the natural log scale, and the transition in the odds of oral cancer between smokers and non-smokers is represented by the two parallel lines. The fact that the lines are parallel demonstrates that the elevated odds of oral cancer from smoking are the same (on the log scale) for both users and non-users of betel nut. However, the estimated odds and odds ratios are different from those observed in Table 8.1. For example, the odds for people who smoke but do not use betel nut are 30/6000 = 0.005, which is lower than the estimated 0.006.

Figure 8.2 shows the observed relationships between oral cancer odds and smoking stratified by the use of betel nut on the log scale, in which the two transition lines between non-smokers and smokers are no longer parallel. To obtain the observed odds for each subgroup, we run a logistic regression with an interaction term that is the product of *smoking* and *betel nut*:

$$\text{logit}(\pi) = -5.81 + 0.511\,\text{smoking} + 0.734\,\text{betelnut} + 0.47\,\text{smoking} * \text{betel nut}. \quad (8.2)$$

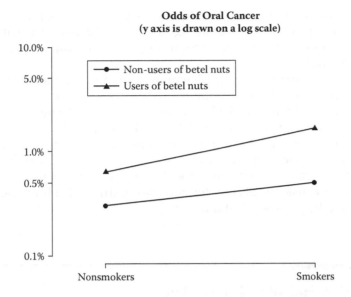

FIGURE 8.2
The relation between the odds of oral cancer and using betel nut in smokers and non-smokers estimated using logistic regression with an interaction term between smoking and the use of betel nut.

We can work out the odds for each subgroup: the odds for smokers without using betel nut is $\exp(-5.81 + 0.511) = 0.005$, the odds for smokers with the use of betel nut is $\exp(-5.81 + 0.511 + 0.734 + 0.47) = 0.0167$, the odds for non-smokers without using betel nut is $\exp(-5.81) = 0.003$, and the odds for non-smokers with the use of betel nut is $\exp(-5.81 + 0.734) = 0.0062$. These figures are now in line with those obtained in Table 8.1.

Therefore, including an interaction term in Equation 8.2 yielded better estimates of the odds (hence prevalence) of oral cancer in each subgroup. As the two lines in Figure 8.2 are diverging, there appears to be a synergistic effect between smoking and using betel nut. On the other hand, with no interaction, as in Equation 8.1, the two lines in Figure 8.1 will always be parallel (on the log scale) because it is assumed that the effect of smoking on the log odds of oral cancer is the same in betel nut users and non-users, and vice versa. However, it should be noted that our hypothetical example is overtly simplistic because the statistical interaction between two exposures is scale dependent; at each stage we have had to labour the scale upon which any interpretation takes place. Consequently, testing statistical interaction is not necessarily equivalent to evaluating and formally testing biological interaction, and the latter is likely to be dose–response dependent. The inclusion of statistical interaction in the model is simply to relax an unnecessary constraint and thereby improve the estimation of cancer prevalence in each subgroup. There is not necessarily any direct interpretation of the statistical interaction to be made, yet many researchers are quite easily distracted by the ease of undertaking such formal evaluation. This is why there is often much confusion surrounding the use of statistical interaction in epidemiology.

In summary, from a statistical viewpoint, including an interaction term in the model is to provide better estimates to the (log) odds (or means when the outcomes are continuous variables in linear regression); there is limited gain in biological understanding from statistical interaction. In our hypothetical example, the interaction term may not be formally statistically significant; that is, the inclusion of this product variable does not significantly improve the model compared to the one without it, but that should not be the basis by which one considers relaxing (or not) the constraint that is implied by the choice of model parameterisation.

8.2 Testing Statistical Interaction between Continuous Variables

Epidemiologists are more familiar with testing statistical interaction between categorical variables, as it appears to be equivalent to estimating means or log odds for each risk subgroup. Therefore, when exposure variables are continuous, a common practice is to divide them into several categories using cut-off values such as median, tertiles or quartiles. The greater the number of categories, the greater the number of product interaction terms generated. As a result, it is not always a useful approach and has its undesired consequences, which will be discussed later in this chapter.

Testing statistical interaction between two continuous variables is technically no different from testing statistical interaction between two categorical variables. A product term is generated between the two continuous covariates and entered into the model. The difficulty becomes how to interpret the regression coefficient for the interaction term or how to interpret the overall model.

It is more convenient to use simulated examples to illustrate statistical interaction between continuous variables. We use software package R to generate two variables x and z:

```
## R codes
> x<-c(10:500)/10 ## x = (1,1.1,1.2...4.9,5)
> z<-5+0.5*x+rnorm(491,0,5) ## z is the sum of x and a random
variable with zero mean and standard deviation equal to 5
```

The total number of observations is 491 and the correlation between x and z is 0.82. We then generate y as a linear combination of x and z plus another random variable:

```
> y<-10+0.3*x+0.6*z+rnorm(491,0,5)
```

If we run a linear regression for *y* regressed on *x* and *z*, the regression coefficients should be close to 0.3 and 0.6, and the intercept close to 10. The edited output from *R* for this linear model (we call it Model 1) is

```
Call:
lm(formula = y ~ x + z) ## y is regressed on x and z
Coefficients:
            Estimate Std. Error t value Pr(>|t|)
(Intercept) 10.35005    0.51481   20.11  <2e-16
x            0.33255    0.02774   11.99  <2e-16
z            0.53290    0.04635   11.50  <2e-16
```

The results are similar to what we set up in the simulation. Figure 8.3a is a three-dimensional scatterplot showing the fitted surface for the predicted values of *y* in Model 1 and the observed data points for *y*. The grid lines in the fitted surface represent the expected increase in *y* when *x* or *z* increases by one unit. For example, the regression coefficient for *x* is 0.33, so when *x* increases by 1, *y* is expected to increase by 0.33 irrespective of the values of *z*; and when *z* increases by 1, *y* is expected to increase by 0.53 irrespective of the values of *x*. All grid lines in the direction *x* have the same slope of 0.33, and grid lines in the direction of *z* have the same slope of 0.53.

We now generate another variable *y*1 as a linear combination of *x*, *z* and the product of *x* and *z*:

```
> y1<-10+0.3*x+0.6*z+0.01*x*z+rnorm(491,0,5)
```

We regress *y*1 on *x* and *z*, and the edited results from R for this model (we call it Model 2) are

```
Call:
lm(formula = y1 ~ x + z)
Coefficients:
            Estimate Std. Error t value Pr(>|t|)
(Intercept)  6.90999    0.53453   12.93  <2e-16
x            0.50624    0.02880   17.58  <2e-16
z            0.78786    0.04812   16.37  <2e-16
```

The fitted surface still looks like a flat surface but with different slopes (Figure 8.3b) from those in Model 1. However, we are missing a covariate in Model 2: the product of *x* and *z*. We now regress *y*1 on *x*, *z* and *x* ∗ *z* (and call it Model 3), and the results from R are

```
Call:
lm(formula = y1 ~ x * z)
```

```
Coefficients:
              Estimate Std. Error t value Pr(>|t|)
(Intercept) 11.210722    0.854412  13.121   < 2e-16
x            0.289091    0.044214   6.538 1.57e-10
z            0.469106    0.068569   6.841 2.36e-11
x*z          0.012502    0.001983   6.305 6.48e-10
```

The product interaction term is highly significant, which should not be a surprise. Figure 8.3c shows the fitted surface for the predicted $y1$ and the observed data points. The main differences between Figures 8.3b and 8.3c are that the plane in Figure 8.3c is slightly twisted toward the larger values of x and z. Therefore, the grid lines in either x or z directions no longer have the same slopes. This can be explained by rearranging the equation for Model 3:

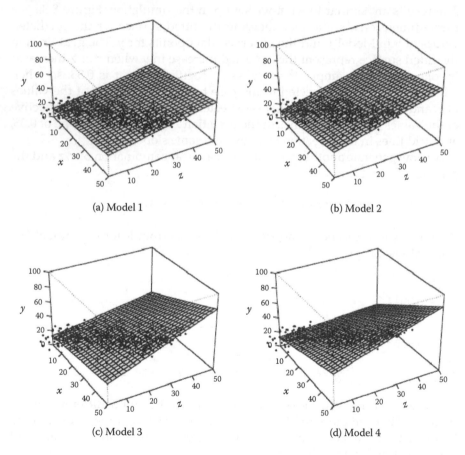

(a) Model 1

(b) Model 2

(c) Model 3

(d) Model 4

FIGURE 8.3
Three-dimensional scatterplots with fitted surfaces for the outcomes. The dots are observed values of the outcomes, and the grid surfaces are the predicted values of the outcomes.

$$y1 = 11.2 + 0.29x + 0.47z + 0.013x*z, \tag{8.3}$$

$$y1 = 11.2 + 0.29x + (0.47 + 0.013x)z, \tag{8.4}$$

$$y1 = 11.2 + (0.29 + 0.013z)x + 0.47z. \tag{8.5}$$

Equations 8.4 and 8.5 show that the slope for x is related to the values of z and the slope for z is related to the values of x. For example, the slope for x is 0.29 when $z = 0$, but 0.42 when $z = 10$; that is, the expected (or predicted) increase in $y1$ when x increases by one unit is dependent upon the level of z. The greater the values of z, the greater the expected increase in $y1$ when x increases by one unit. Suppose $y1$ is blood pressure (*BP*), x body mass index (BMI) and z-ages. Model 3 suggests that the impact of obesity on *BP* depend on people's age, and we may interpret this result as an interaction between BMI and ages (on the respective scales of kg/m^2 and years).

We now generate a new variable $y2$ that has a rather complex relation with x and z:

```
## R code
> x2<-x^2    ## x2 is squared x
> y2<-10+0.3*x+0.6*z+0.01*x2+rnorm(491,0,5)
```

Note that the product term $x*z$ was not used in generating $y2$; instead, we assume a quadratic relationship between $y2$ and x conditional on z. However, suppose we do not know the correct relationship (i.e., correct underlying model), so we mistakenly regress $y2$ on x, z and $x*z$ (Model 4):

```
Call:
lm(formula = y2 ~ x * z)
Coefficients:
             Estimate Std. Error t value Pr(>|t|)
(Intercept) 11.124424   0.869081  12.800  < 2e-16 ***
x            0.585259   0.044974  13.013  < 2e-16 ***
z            0.135048   0.069746   1.936   0.0534 .
x*z          0.015144   0.002017   7.509 2.87e-13 ***
```

Results from Model 4 shows that the interaction term is highly significant, and the fitted surface is shown in Figure 8.3(d). The difficulty is in knowing if Model 4 is a wrong model and the interaction is spurious or not. In empirical research, it is hard to make a judgment because we rarely know the correct mathematical underlying relationships between the outcome and all covariates. When the correct relation between y and covariates is specified, the interaction is no longer significant (Model 5):

```
## Edited R output
Call:
lm(formula = y2 ~ x * z + x2)
Coefficients:
              Estimate Std. Error t value Pr(>|t|)
(Intercept) 11.198137   0.855029  13.097  < 2e-16
x            0.332282   0.075130   4.423 1.20e-05
z            0.420390   0.096943   4.336 1.76e-05
x2           0.008542   0.002050   4.166 3.67e-05
x*z          0.004346   0.003264   1.331    0.184
```

In summary, our simulations illustrate that, from a statistical point of view, testing interaction is just to fit different relationships between the outcome and covariates. A significant interaction suggests that a more complex surface or plane seems to provide a better approximation to the observed data. Interpreting statistical interaction as biological interaction, however, is only feasible when the underlying relationship between the outcome and covariates are simple and the scale upon which they are modelled is clearly interpretable in biological terms.

8.3 Partial Regression Coefficient for Product Term in Regression Models

In this section we discuss testing interaction between continuous variables from a theoretical perspective. Suppose y is a continuous outcome variable, x is the exposure, z is an effect modifier, and xz is the product term derived from x multiplied by z. The multiple linear regression model is expressed as

$$y = b_0 + b_1 x + b_2 z + b_3 xz + \varepsilon, \tag{8.6}$$

where b_0 is the intercept, b_1 is the partial regression coefficient for x, b_2 is the partial regression coefficient for z, b_3 the partial regression coefficient for xz, and ε is the random error term in the model. If the three continuous variables y, x, and z follow a multivariate normal distribution, it can be shown that the expected value of b_3 is zero irrespective of the bivariate correlations amongst y, x and z. The mathematical proof can be found in our previous publication (Tu et al. 2007).

Testing product terms, such as xz, in a linear regression has been proposed as a test to examine the *linearity* and *multivariate normality* of continuous variables (Cox and Small 1978; Cox and Wermuth 1994), as multivariate normality requires that (a) all marginal distributions are normal (e.g., each variable is normally distributed) and (b) the relationships amongst the variables are linear. The latter point indicates that the interaction effect is scale dependent, and nonlinear transformations of the original variables (such as log-transformation) might attenuate an interaction effect or even produce a non-zero interaction effect were it is zero on the original scale. For example, if we take the natural log-transformation for x (*lnx*) in Model 1 in Section 8.2, and run a linear regression for y on lnx and z:

```
Call:
lm(formula = y ~ lnx * z)
Coefficients:
            Estimate Std. Error t value Pr(>|t|)
(Intercept) 12.03995    1.46170   8.237 1.64e-15
lnx          1.53267    0.55146   2.779 0.00566
z           -0.21006    0.14205  -1.479 0.13985
lnx*z        0.26366    0.03949   6.676 6.71e-11
```

Whilst there is no statistical interaction between x and z in the original model, the product interaction term is now statistically significant. Figure 8.4 shows the scatterplot for y, lnx and z. So suppose y is blood pressure, x is BMI and z is age. Can we conclude that although there is no synergistic effect of BMI and age on *BP*, there is evidence to suggest that there is synergistic effect of log BMI and age on *BP*? Many exposure variables are nonlinearly transformed first before being used for regression modelling to correct for their

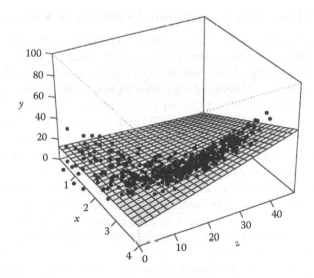

FIGURE 8.4
Three-dimensional scatterplots with fitted surfaces for the outcome. The dots are observed values of the outcome, and the grid surfaces are the predicted values of the outcome. One covariate (*lnx*) has been transformed using natural log.

skewed distributions. This example illustrates the potential caveats in this approach to test statistical interaction.

From a geometrical viewpoint, if the three continuous variables y, x and z follow a multivariate normal distribution, the data points configure an ellipsoid (in three-dimensional space). Regressing y on x and z simultaneously is equivalent to fitting a plane to the data (as shown in Figure 8.3). Therefore, incorporating the product interaction term xz in Equation 8.6 amounts to testing whether or not the fitted plane is flat (equivalent to a zero xz regression coefficient, such as those in Figures 8.3a and 8.3b) or twisted (non-zero coefficient, such as those in Figures 8.3c, 8.3d and 8.4). Owing to multivariate normality, the best-fitting plane using ordinary least-squares should be perfectly flat.

From a statistical viewpoint, some epidemiologists and statisticians might consider the finding that the expected value of the partial regression coefficient for xz is zero under multivariate normality to be inconsequential since the assumption of multivariate normality requires that all marginal distributions are normal, and this might therefore be only an extreme case. However, the implication of this finding in epidemiological research is far from trivial, as will be demonstrated in the following section.

8.4 Categorization of Continuous Explanatory Variables

It is not uncommon in epidemiology that continuous explanatory variables are divided into two or more groups because researchers might believe that (1) it is easier to interpret the results of categorical variables, (2) effect size can be maximised in categorical variables (Altman 1994; Altman et al. 1994; Wartenberg and Northridge 1994), or (3) the relation between the outcome and explanatory variable is not linear (Wartenberg and Northridge 1994). It is well known that categorization of the continuous explanatory variable will reduce the statistical power to detect its relation with the outcome (Cox 1957; Zhao and Kolonel 1992; MacCallum et al. 2002), and sometimes this can give rise to biased estimates of the effect size of an exposure variable when a continuous confounding variable is categorised (Cumsille et al. 2000; Taylor and Yu 2002). However, categorisation can also be viewed as a nonlinear transformation like the log transformation in Section 8.3 for variable x, and it may give rise to misleading results.

The consequence of categorising exposure and/or effect modifier on the detection and estimation of the interaction is relatively unknown in the epidemiological literature. Therefore, we use the foetal origins of adult disease hypothesis (see Chapter 7) to illustrate the possible consequence of categorising continuous explanatory variables in a multiple linear regression model.

8.5 The Four-Model Principle in the Foetal Origins Hypothesis

In a widely discussed article, Lucas et al. (1999) proposed a four-model principle to test the foetal origins of adult disease hypothesis. Suppose an epidemiological study would like to test whether or not birth weight (BW) is a risk factor of higher blood pressure (BP) in later life, whilst also considering current body weight (CW). Lucas et al. argued that results from the following four models should be tested and presented:

Model 1 (early model): $BP = a_1 + b_1 BW$,

Model 2 (later model): $BP = a_2 + c_2 CW$,

Model 3 (combined model): $BP = a_3 + b_3 BW + c_3 CW$,

Model 4 (interaction model): $BP = a_4 + b_4 BW + c_4$current body weight + $d_4 BW * CW$,

where $BW * CW$ is a product interaction term derived by multiplying BW by CW. Lucas et al. (1999) suggested that b_1, b_3, b_4 and d_4 are expected to be negative in support of the foetal origins hypothesis. In the previous literature, b_1 is often very close to zero or weakly negative. However, b_3 is usually negative and statistically significant due to the adjustment for current body weight in the combined model, although it has been argued that this is a result of over-adjustment (Paneth and Susser 1995; Paneth et al. 1996) and might suffer the statistical artifact known as the *reversal paradox* (see Chapter 7). Lucas et al. (1999) used their data on log insulin concentration in 358 children aged 9–12 years, who had been born prematurely, to test these models; they found that the partial regression coefficient for the product interaction term in Model 4 was positive though not significant (0.028; 95% CI = −0.001, 0.057).

Since then, a few studies have applied the four-model principle in their regression modelling to test the foetal origins hypothesis. In a study on systolic BP in children aged 11–12 years, Walker et al. (2001) found the interaction between birth weight and current body weight to be −0.62 (95% CI = −1.52, 0.29). In another study on blood pressure in children and young adults (Williams and Poulton 2002), the interaction between current body weight and either birth weight or birth length were negative, though without statistical significance. In a study on systolic blood pressure, Burke et al. (2004) found that the interaction between birth weight and current body weight, and between birth length and current height, were both negative though very close to zero and without statistical significance. In a recent large study on total cholesterol concentration by Davies et al. (2004), no significant interaction between birth weight and current body mass index (BMI) was found in either men or women; partial regression coefficients for the interaction terms were −0.001 (95% CI = −0.008, 0.007) for men and −0.004 (95% CI = −0.01, 0.005) for women.

It seems to appear that no study on the foetal origins hypothesis has yet reported a negative and statistically significant d_4 using Model 4 (the interaction model). However, this might not be too surprising were blood pressure (or any continuous health outcome), birth weight and current body weight all to follow multivariate normality, as the expected d_4 will be then zero, as shown in the previous section. In the paper by Lucas et al. (1999), the outcome is log-transformed insulin, and they might undertake the transformation for insulin due to its distribution being not normal. It is interesting to know whether the interaction between *BW* and *CW* would become bigger, or even statistically significant, if insulin (instead of log-transformed insulin) had been used as the outcome. When a continuous outcome does not have a normal distribution, researchers tend to undertake a suitable transformation in order that the residual error term (not the continuous outcome per se) is normally distributed.

8.6 Categorization of Continuous Covariates and Testing Interaction

8.6.1 Simulations

To explore the consequences of categorising birth weight and/or current body weight on the estimation of d_4 in the interaction model, we conducted computer simulations in our previous study (Tu et al. 2007). The design of these simulations was based on the four-model principle for the foetal origin hypothesis, such that synthetic data were generated for a hypothetical sample of 30-year-old adult males for three variables: current systolic blood pressure, birth weight and current body weight. Mean values and their standard deviations were derived from the literature (Hennessy and Alberman 1998) and from the results of surveys conducted by the UK Department of Health in 2002 for adult males aged 26 to 34 (http://www.doh.gov.uk): *BW* = 3.38 kg (SD = 0.57 kg); *BP* = 129.0 mmHg (SD = 12.3 mmHg); *CW* = 83.0 kg (SD = 16.1 kg). The function **mvrnorm** in the MASS package (Ripley and Venables 2002) in *R* was used to generate the trivariate normal data.

Three alternative scenarios were simulated: (1) no relationship between *BW* and *BP* (i.e., the Pearson correlation, *r*, between *BW* and *BP* was zero); (2) a modest *inverse* relationship between *BW* and *BP* (i.e., *r* between *BW* and *BP* was −0.1); and (3) a modest *positive* relationship between *BW* and *BP* (i.e., *r* between *BW* and *BP* was +0.1). The pairwise correlations of *BW*, *BP*, and *CW* in each of the scenarios just outlined were simulated for correlations with a range of different values. The correlations between *BP* and *BW*, and between *BP* and *CW* were *r* = 0.2 or 0.4. The choice of correlation values adopted was motivated by typical values encountered within the literature (see Chapter 7).

Our simulations showed that when BW and/or CW were categorised by their medians, the type-I error rates were still close to the nominal 5%. However, when they were categorised according to the 25th percentile or 75th percentile, probabilities of detecting an interaction increases with sample size. In the sample of 20,000 subjects, the type-I error rate sometimes got close to 50%. Inflated type-I error rates occurred when BW and CW were categorised by their tertiles, quartiles or quintiles; that is, they were divided into groups with equal number of observations. However, the probabilities of detecting an interaction also increased with sample size. The greatest type-I error rates were around 40%, 30% and 20%, when BW and CW were categorised using tertiles, quartiles, or quintiles, respectively. The probabilities of detecting the interaction were thus dependent on the number of categories and increased as the number of categories declined. This is because the greater the number of balanced groups into which the original variables were categorised, the greater resemblance the categorised variables bore to the original continuous variables. Just as with histograms, the smaller the category width, the more similar the histograms look like a normal curve.

Further simulations showed that when BW and CW were categorised according to some predefined values, yielding unequal observations in the categorical variables, the probabilities of detecting statistical interaction could be as high as 99%. This is because the categorisation caused nonlinear transformations of original variables, giving rise to spurious statistical interaction.

8.6.2 Numerical Example

A previously common practice in epidemiological research in the foetal origins hypothesis was to categorise BW and CW into several groups, and then the mean values of the outcome variable are calculated for each cell in a contingency table. For instance, subjects are grouped by their BW and CW, where both variables are categorised into five categories. Either the mean BP or the percentage of the subjects with BP greater than a threshold value is then calculated for each subgroup (forming a 5×5 table). Consequently, a trend might be observed where subjects with lower BW but higher CW have greater BP and increased risk of hypertension. This practice can be potentially misleading because it is comparable to testing the interaction between these two variables. For illustration, a sample of 5000 subjects was generated using the parameters in scenario 1. The mean values of BP, BW and CW were 129.1 mmHg (SD = 12.3 mmHg), 3.4 kg (SD = 0.57 kg) and 83.2 kg (SD = 16.1 kg), respectively. The correlation between BP and BW was 0.001, the correlation between BP and CW was 0.299, and the correlation between CW and BW was 0.201. The partial regression coefficient for the product term in the interaction model (Model 4 in the four models proposed by Lucas et al. 1999) was −0.002 ($P = 0.931$), indicating that there was no statistical interaction effect. However, when *BW* was categorised into five categories (<2.5, 2.5 to 3, 3 to 3.5, 3.5 to 4, >4) and *CW* was also categorised into five categories (<67, 67 to 76, 76 to 85, 85 to 94, >94), the mean *BP* in a 5 × 5 table (Table 8.2) suggested that there was a trend across the stratum where subjects who were born small but grew larger had a greater mean *BP* and a greater risk of hypertension (defined as *BP* > 135 mmHg). In contrast, subjects born larger who grew smaller had a lower mean *BP* and a lower risk of hypertension. Logistic regression with categorised *BW* and *CW* and their 16 product terms on the risk of hypertension shows that the *P*-value for the overall interaction effect was 0.015. As there is no evidence of a statistical interaction between *BW* and *CW* on *BP* in the logistic regression with original continuous variables, the impression that subjects with low *BW* but high *CW* (known as catch-up growth) have greater risk of hypertension is spurious and potentially misleading.

8.7 Discussion

Our simulation study showed that when the three continuous variables (the outcome, exposure and effect modifier) follow multivariate normality, dichotomising both the exposure, *BW*, and effect modifier, *CW*, using values other than their medians (which are equivalent to the means since they all follow normal distribution) might give rise to a spurious statistical interaction effect in regression analysis. When *BW* and *CW* were categorised into two groups using thresholds other than their medians, the partial regression coefficient for the product interaction term departed from the expected value of zero, and the type-I error rates became inflated. Therefore, a spurious statistical interaction between *BW* and *CW* in terms of their effects on *BP* might be detected, whilst in reality there was none. The departure from zero and the type-I error rates became greater when the correlations or sample sizes increased. If *BW* and *CW* were categorised into multiple groups, the type-I error rates exceeded 5%, where *BW* and *CW* were categorised into multiple groups with equal number of subjects in each groups using tertiles, quartiles or quintiles values, or into multiple groups with unequal number of subjects in each group using predefined thresholds. Simulations demonstrated that the practice of categorising continuous explanatory variables to test their statistical interaction is questionable and may potentially yield misleading results. Therefore, one common practice of testing the heterogeneity of the relationship between the outcome and exposure by evaluating their relation in each stratum of a categorised continuous effect modifier is potentially misleading. This practice usually aims to identify subgroups of subjects who might be more responsive to the exposure, though this could be misguided.

TABLE 8.2

Tabulation of A Hypothetical Data Generated Using the Parameters in Scenario One

Current Body Weight (kg)		Birth Weight (kg)					
		<2.5	≥2.5 & <3	≥3 & <3.5	≥3.5 & <4	≥4	All
<67	Blood pressure (mmHg)	124.9	123.9	124.3	122.7	121.1	123.7
	% Hypertension	18	17	19	16	12	17
	Number of subjects	80	167	295	172	65	779
≥67 & <76	Blood pressure (mmHg)	128.6	127.1	126.4	125.0	125.7	126.3
	% Hypertension	35	23	24	19	20	23
	Number of subjects	71	175	297	218	87	848
≥76 & <85	Blood pressure (mmHg)	129.6	128.2	128.4	128.4	126.0	128.1
	% Hypertension	28	27	28	30	18	27
	Number of subjects	71	224	350	292	148	1,085
≥85 & <94	Blood pressure (mmHg)	131.7	131.3	130.4	130.4	130.5	130.6
	% Hypertension	43	36	33	35	32	34
	Number of subjects	42	154	362	303	169	1,030
≥94	Blood pressure (mmHg)	130.8	135.4	134.7	133.6	132.2	128.7
	% Hypertension	38	53	49	43	42	46
	Number of subjects	47	169	384	406	252	1,258
All	Blood pressure (mmHg)	128.6	129.1	129.2	129.1	128.7	129.1
	% Hypertension	31	31	32	31	29	31
	Number of subjects	311	889	1,688	1,391	721	5,000

Note: Although there is no interaction between birth weight (BW) and current body weight (CW) between the original continuous variables, the 5 × 5 table according to categorised BW and CW seems to show that subjects who were born small but grow larger have higher mean blood pressure (BP) and greater risk of hypertension (i.e., BP > 135 mmHg), and the subjects who were born larger but grow smaller have lower mean BP and lower risk of hypertension.

In our simulation study (Tu et al. 2007), CW was chosen as the effect modifier and it was assumed that BP, BW and CW all follow multivariate normal distribution. Suppose an additional effect modifier, current body height (CH), also follows multivariate normality, then the statistical interaction between BW and CH within a regression model is also zero. Using body mass index ($BMI = CW/CH^2$) as the effect modifier instead of CW or CH, the three variables, BP, BW and BMI, may no longer be multivariate normal because the relation between BP and BMI, or between BW and BMI, might not be linear. Consequently, a spurious statistical interaction between BW and BMI might be detected. Therefore, Lucas et al. (1999) were right to argue that BMI should be avoided when testing the interaction model.

Although Lucas et al. (1999) proposed the four-model principle to test the foetal origins hypothesis, they did not postulate a biological theory to explain their statistical models. They argued that the partial regression coefficient (d_4) should be negative if the foetal origins hypothesis is true. The Model 4 in their paper can be rearranged as

Model 4 (interaction model): $BP = a_4 + b_4 BW + (c_4 + d_4 BW) * CW$.

Therefore, a negative d_4 would mean that the positive relation between BP and CW is not homogeneous across all levels of birth weight. In particular, for people born larger, increased BP due to increased adult body weight per 1 kg is less than that in people born smaller. In other words, the 'adverse' impact of increased adult body weight is greater in people born smaller than those born larger. Since the publication of the four-model principle, several more complex and sophisticated statistical models have been proposed to test the foetal origins hypothesis, and we shall discuss some of them in Chapters 9 and 10.

The implications from this chapter are much broader for epidemiology than we have alluded to by using the foetal origins hypothesis for the purpose of illustration. For instance, testing statistical interaction plays a very important role in finding gene–environment interactions; that is, how the effects of genes (which is not manipulable) on the risk of disease are affected by environmental exposures (which in theory can be controlled). Therefore, prevention measures can be specifically designed and implemented for those with the greatest need. However, as our illustrations show, the transformation of variables involved may change the results of statistical testing of product interaction terms. Suppose the research question is to know whether there is an interaction between one genetic polymorphism and obesity on blood insulin level, and whether the regression coefficient for the product term between binary genetic polymorphism and continuous body weight is close to zero. Does this mean that there is no biological interaction? What if we log-transform the outcome insulin and find that the regression coefficient for the product term is no longer zero and statistically significant?

Another even more complex scenario is where the relationships between an outcome and several explanatory variables are not linear, as shown in Section 8.3. For instance, in our example of insulin, genes and obesity, suppose the relationship between insulin and *BW* is curvilinear but we erroneously specify a linear relationship within our regression model without incorporating, say, a quadratic term for *BW*. We may then detect a statistical interaction between the genetic polymorphism and *BW*, but, in fact, what we should have done is to specify a curvilinear relationship, and no such statistical interaction would have occurred. Our biological interpretation of the two potential models could then seem contradictory, and this highlights the difficulty in projecting a biological interpretation of interaction onto what is observed as statistical interaction.

8.8 Conclusion

When blood pressure, birth weight and current body weight follow multivariate normality, the expected value of the partial regression coefficient for the statistical interaction between birth weight and current body weight is zero, irrespective of the bivariate correlations amongst these three variables (Tu et al. 2007). In the foetal origins hypothesis, birth size and current body size are often categorised to create a contingency table. However, when birth weight and current body weight are categorised, a spurious statistical interaction effect might be observed, and false-positive error rates increase as the sample size and/or the variable correlations increase. An important implication is that testing statistical interaction is scale dependent, whereas biological interaction is not; hence there is not always a clear link between the statistical and biological interpretations of interaction. Without a clear theory of biological interaction, testing statistical interaction is subject to many different interpretations.

9

Finding Growth Trajectories in Lifecourse Research

9.1 Introduction

In Chapters 7 and 8 we have discussed several statistical models for testing associations between birth size and chronic diseases in later life, known as the foetal origins of adult disease hypothesis (FOAD) or Barker's hypothesis. This hypothesis has attracted considerable attention amongst the medical and epidemiological research communities over the last two decades. In the previous chapters we also showed that the associations between birth size and chronic diseases can often be weak (negative or positive) but then become negative and statistically significant when current body size is adjusted for in the model as a covariate. In recent years, attention to the foetal origins hypothesis has gradually shifted from birth size to early postnatal growth, and it has been suggested that small birth size in conjunction with compensatory rapid growth in childhood (rather than small birth size per se) might lead to a greater risk of developing chronic adult diseases. As a result, the FOAD hypothesis has been rephrased *the developmental origins of health and disease hypothesis* (DOHaD hypothesis; Barker 2004; Barker et al. 2005; Gillman 2005). In fact, both FOAD and DOHaD may be viewed as members of a larger theme, that of lifecourse epidemiology, in which researchers are interested in 'the study of long-term effects on chronic disease risk of physical and social exposures during gestation, childhood, adolescence, young adulthood and later adult life' (Ben-Shlomo and Kuh 2002). Lifecourse epidemiology involves studies of the 'biological, behavioural and psychosocial pathways that operate across an individual's lifecourse, as well as across generations, to influence the development of chronic diseases' (Ben-Shlomo and Kuh 2002).

Several recent articles have presented evidence that people who develop adult chronic diseases, such as coronary heart disease (Eriksson et al. 2000, 2001; Forsen et al. 2004; Barker et al. 2005) and diabetes (Eriksson et al. 2003a, 2003b; Bhargava et al. 2004), tend to have had a distinct growth trajectory. Using z-scores to track relative body sizes over time, it has been shown that individuals who developed chronic adult diseases have also had, on average, below-average birth size and low weight during infancy. These people remained smaller in their early childhood but started to catch up and gain weight rapidly as they grew older. By the time of puberty, their body weight (BW) and body mass index (BMI) exceeds the average for their age. Whilst tracking the growth trajectories using body size z-scores seems to be a straightforward approach, the apparent association of accelerated growth with the risk of chronic diseases in later life may be in part or entirely due to the well-known statistical phenomenon of regression to the mean. In the next section we use an example to illustrate the potential difficulties in interpreting z-score growth trajectories.

9.1.1 Example: Catch-Up Growth and Impaired Glucose Tolerance

Our example uses data kindly made available by Professor Clive Osmond at the University of Southampton, UK, on his website (http://www.mrc.soton.ac.uk/index.asp?page=87), and this data set had been made public for a conference of the Developmental Origins of Health and Disease Society in Toronto (2005). In the data set, the body weight of 1000 men was measured at birth, at least twice or more before the age of 10 years, and again at 30 years. Figure 9.1 displays the growth trajectory between birth and the age of 10 years for men who subsequently developed impaired glucose tolerance (IGT; defined as > 7.0 mmole per litre) by the age of 30 years. The plot is of their average z-score weights at each age (z-scores were derived by subtracting the mean weight of the whole group at that age from the individual weights, then dividing by the standard deviation for the whole group at that age).

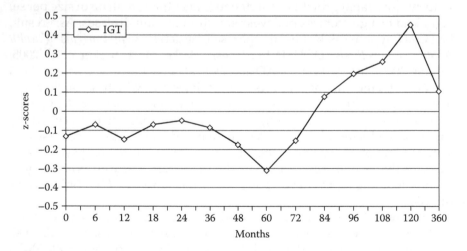

FIGURE 9.1
Mean z-scores for body weight from birth to the age of 30 years for men who developed impaired glucose tolerance (IGT) by the age of 30.

Before the age of 7 years, the mean z-score weight of men with IGT was negative; that is, below the average (which is zero by definition): this group achieved above-average body weight at the age of 8 years. After 8 years, men with IGT gained more weight than those with normal glucose tolerance. According to the DOHaD hypothesis (Barker 2004; Gillman 2005), and as reported in a number of studies (Eriksson et al. 2003a, 2003b; Bhargava et al. 2004), this indicates that compensatory growth in body weight during childhood is associated with the risk of developing abnormal glucose tolerance in later life.

If there is an association between catch-up growth and the risk of developing chronic adult diseases, then tracking children's early growth trajectory might provide a means to identify those children who might develop chronic diseases in later life and therefore facilitate the implementation of prevention programmes at an early age. However, the apparent evidence of the association between growth trajectories and adult disease displayed in graphs such as Figure 9.1 may be explained by the well-known statistical phenomenon of regression to the mean. Although there are many discussions of this phenomenon in the medical and epidemiological literature, most pertain to the comparison of changes between two treatment groups (often in a pre-test/post-test study design; for example, see Chapter 4).

9.1.2 Galton and Regression to the Mean

In our short historical review of regression to the mean in Chapter 4, we mentioned that Galton was an important figure in the eugenic movement in nineteenth century Britain (Stigler 1997; Senn 2003; Hanley 2004; Gillham 2009) and that he was interested in the inheritance of human intelligence. As there were no reliable measures for intelligence, he turned to human body measurements and collected self-reported body heights from families. As men were on average taller than women, women's heights were multiplied by 1.08. Galton (1886) then investigated the correlation between the average of both parents' heights (he called it mid-parent height) and the heights of their adult children by subtracting the mean from each individual height. Galton found that although children of tall parents were still taller than most people, they were on average shorter than their parents. On the other hand, adult children of short parents, whilst still short, were on average taller than their parents.

Discussions in the medical and statistical literature have tended to overlook an important subtlety in Galton's body heights example. Examining his data in reverse time order, Galton's data also show that parents of tall children were on average shorter than their children, and parents of short children were on average taller than their parents. In Galton's data, the average height of both parents and their children was around 68 inches, so we transform the raw height measurements into sample z-scores for both parents and children, as we did previously. Figure 9.2 shows the trend of body

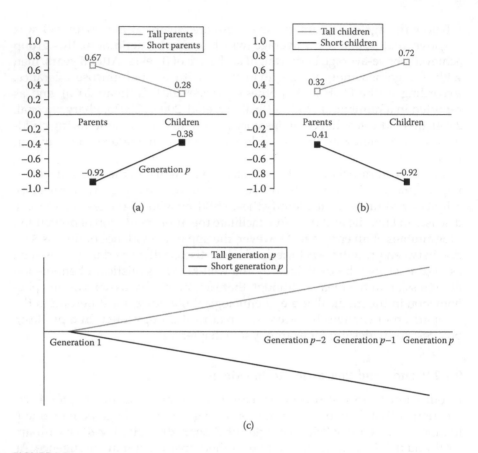

FIGURE 9.2
Trend in body height across generations: (a) mean body height of subgroups in Galton's data when the families are grouped by parents' height or (b) by children's height; (c) evolution of body height throughout many generations when families were grouped by the height of the youngest generation (generation *p*).

height *z*-scores across two generations using Galton's data (Galton 1886). In Figure 9.2a, families are grouped according to the parents' heights by defining parents as tall or short according to whether their average height was greater or less than 68 inches. The mean height *z*-scores of tall and short parents were 0.67 and −0.92, respectively. The mean body height *z*-score of adult children from tall parents was 0.28 and that of adult children from short parents was −0.38. Therefore, human heights appear to be converging across the two generations, suggesting that, after many generations, there would be fewer very tall or very short people, whilst the average height remains constant. Figure 9.2b shows an apparently contradictory trend of body heights across the two generations by grouping the families according to adult children's heights. Children were defined as tall or short according to whether their height was greater or equal to or less than 68 in.: mean height z-scores in these groups were 0.72 and –0.92. The mean height z-score of parents of tall children was 0.32 and that of parents of short children was –0.41. Therefore, human heights appear to be diverging, so that after several generations there might be very tall or very short people although the average height remains stable.

In fact, neither of these two contradictory interpretations of Galton's data is correct. The patterns in Figures 9.2a and 9.2b are consequences of the correlation between the heights of parents and their children not being perfect (i.e., less than 1). Regression to the mean occurs either when children's heights are regressed on their parents' heights, or vice versa; in either case the regression coefficient is less than unity.

Now consider the trend that Galton would have observed if he had obtained records of body heights of grandparents for his families. If families were grouped according to the youngest generation's heights, the converging trend of human body heights would become even more apparent, while in contrast if families were grouped according to the oldest generation's heights, the diverging trend would look more evident. The phenomenon of regression to the mean becomes more notable than in Figures 9.2a and 9.2b because the correlation between the heights of grandparents and grandchildren is smaller than between the grandparents and parents, or between the parents and children.

If there was a long historical record of body heights for these families, what might the evolution of human body heights throughout several generations look like? If the families were grouped according to the heights of the last generation, the two diverging lines of human body heights would look like those in Figure 9.2c; the resemblance of ancestors and descendants would diminish with time. Our appearance and characteristics are more similar to that of our parents than our grandparents, and our resemblance to our ancestors diminishes further with each generation. Eventually, our ancestors will be no more like us than an average person in their generation. In his seminal paper in 1886, Galton explained: 'The child inherits partly from his parents, partly from his ancestry. Speaking generally, the further his genealogy goes back, the more numerous and varied will his ancestry become, until they cease to differ from any equally numerous sample taken at haphazard from the race at large. Their mean stature will then be the same as that of the race; in other words, it will be mediocre' (Galton 1886, p. 252).

From a statistical viewpoint, positive correlations between body heights of successive generations become smaller the farther back the genealogy goes; as a result, the phenomenon of regression to the mean becomes more noticeable. Figure 9.3 is a generalization of regression to the mean between ancestors' heights and descendants' heights when the data are grouped according to whether the descendant's height is above or below the sample mean (as with Galton's data). When the correlation between ancestors' and descendants' height is perfect and positive (i.e., one), the two lines depicting trajectories are parallel (Figure 9.3a). When the correlation lies between 0 and 1, body heights appear to diverge (Figure 9.3b). When the correlation is

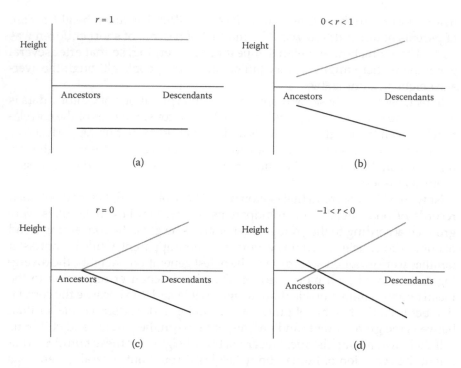

FIGURE 9.3
Generalization of regression to the mean between two variables: X_1—ancestors; X_2—descendants. (a) When the correlation (r) between X_i and X_2 is 1, the two lines depicting the trends are parallel. (b) When r is between 1 and 0, the two lines are diverging. (c) When r is zero, there is no difference in X_1. (d) When r is between 0 and –1, th two lines not only diverge but also cross.

0, there is no difference in mean ancestral height between the two groups (Figure 9.3c). When the correlation is negative, not only do body heights appear to be diverging but the two lines cross (Figure 9.3d).

In summary, when correlated pairs of measurements are grouped according to the value of the later measurement, apparent trajectories in the measurements will be observed when the mean value in each group is plotted against time. The direction of these apparent trajectories depends on the correlation between the measurements and upon which of the data pairs the data is divided.

9.1.3 Revisiting the Growth Trajectory of Men with Impaired Glucose Tolerance

We can now provide a more appropriate interpretation of the patterns of growth observed in men who developed IGT by the age of 30 years. Plotting the mean z-scores of subjects selected because of their adverse health outcomes, as in Figure 9.1, makes the phenomenon of regression to the mean less

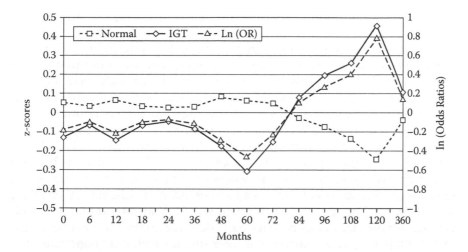

FIGURE 9.4
Mean z-score for body weight from birth to the age of 30 years for men with normal (Normal) or impaired glucose tolerance (IGT) by the age of 30; the natural log of odds ratio (ln(OR)) of developing IGT for per 1 kg increase in body weight at each age is also shown.

recognisable. In Figure 9.4, growth patterns of men with both normal and abnormal glucose tolerance are presented. When the mean weight z-score of one subgroup is less than zero, the mean weight z-score of the other group must by definition be greater than zero, as the average weight z-score of the whole group at each age is zero. If the two groups (normal and IGT) had the same number of subjects and all subjects were measured at identical ages, the two growth trajectories would be perfect mirror images of each other, reflected about the zero axis. Since there are more men with normal than with abnormal glucose tolerance, and not all men were measured at each age, the two patterns of growth in Figure 9.4 are not an exact mirror image, though opposite trends are still evident.

Using our understanding of regression to the mean described in the previous section, the correct interpretation of Figure 9.4 is as follows. Birth weight has an inverse association with IGT, and this inverse association with body weight persists until the age of 6 years. When the two patterns of growth cross, between the ages of 6 and 7 years, the average z-score in each group equals zero; the association of body weight at this age with IGT at 30 years is zero. After the age of 7 years, the association between body weight and IGT becomes positive, and is at its greatest at the age of 10 years. The greater the association (positive or negative) between body weight at a particular age and the adult health outcome, the more separation occurs between the mean z-scores in the two groups.

Figure 9.4 also displays the natural log of the odds ratios (ln(OR)) for the association of body weight at each age with IGT at age 30. Since the difference between the mean z-scores in the two groups reflects the strength of the association, the growth pattern of men with IGT is similar to the trend in the values of the log odds ratio.

In summary, although patterns such as those displayed in Figures 9.1 and 9.4 have been interpreted as growth trajectories, they are better understood as a connected series of cross-sectional associations of body weight at successive ages with IGT at age 30. Substantial upward or downward slopes in these 'trajectories' therefore reflect ages during which the magnitude of the association of body weight with IGT in adulthood is changing rapidly.

Grouping individuals according to their health outcomes in later life is comparable to grouping Galton's families by the children's heights because the outcome (IGT) is most strongly associated with current or the most recent body weight measurement—this is a form of *indirect* mathematical coupling (see Chapter 4). The apparent catch-up growth in mean z-scores for men with IGT does *not* provide evidence that small body size in conjunction with catch-up growth is the *cause* of diabetes in later life. Instead, it demonstrates that birth weight tends to be negatively correlated with adult health outcomes, whilst weight in later childhood tends to be positively correlated; just as the diverging trend in body heights across generations in Galton's families when grouped by children's heights did not mean there would be more and more tall and short people. Confusion arises following the implicit conditioning of the outcome data into groups (normal and IGT) *a priori* to any exploration of the body weight z-scores. The interpretation of Figure 9.1 and similar graphs is therefore conditional on the outcome (disease status), which seriously affects any meaningful inference that is sought of the lifecourse trajectories, though this potential problem is all too frequently overlooked.

9.2 Current Approaches to Identifying Postnatal Growth Trajectories in Lifecourse Research

Apart from tracking body size z-scores, several other approaches have been proposed in recent years to identify the critical growth phases or distinctive growth trajectories that are associated with increased risk of developing chronic diseases in later life. In this section we provide a concise review of such approaches and use an example to compare results. Our data come from a prospective study whose participants were recruited from Metropolitan Cebu, an area of the central Philippines (Adair 2007). Data were obtained from the website of the University of North Carolina Population Centre (http://www.cpc.unc.edu/projects/cebu/datasets.html) and a detailed description of the study can be found on their website and within studies published by Professor Linda Adair and her colleagues (Adair 2007; Dahley et al. 2009). In brief, all pregnant residents of 33 randomly selected Metro

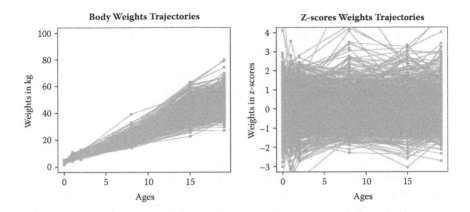

FIGURE 9.5
Observed individual growth trajectories during birth to age 19 years in 834 Cebu girls.

Cebu communities were invited to participate, and index-child participants include 3080 singletons born during a 1-year period beginning April 1983. Prenatal data were collected during the 6 to 7 months of pregnancy.

In this section we use postnatal data of body weights measured immediately after birth, aged 1 year, 2 years, 8 years, 15 years and 19 years. The later-life health outcomes considered are average systolic blood pressure (*SBP*) measured at age 19 years. Raw body weights are transformed to obtain gender-specific z-scores by subtracting sample average weights from individual weights and dividing by sample standard deviations at each age, and participants without complete data are excluded from the sample. In our illustration, we use 834 girls without any missing measurements of body weight or blood pressure for the statistical analyses. Growth in body weight is defined as the change in weight z-scores between consecutive measurements; for example, growth in body weight between birth and age 1 ($zwt_{1-0} = zwt_1 - zwt_0$) is the difference in weight z-scores between birth (zwt_0) and age at 1 yr (zwt_1). Figure 9.5 is the observed growth trajectories for raw body weights and z-score weights between birth and 19 years in 834 Cebu girls. Table 9.1 is a summary of body size measurements and *SBP*.

9.2.1 The Lifecourse Plot

The lifecourse plot is a relatively simple approach proposed by Professor Tim Cole (Cole 2004) from the Institute of Child Health, UK, to identify the critical postnatal growth phases. The outcome variable is regressed on the body size z-scores measured during the early lifecourse using multiple regression, and then the partial regression coefficients for body size z-scores are plotted as a connected line against the ages at which they were measured. The sudden change in the multiple regression coefficients indicates the critical phase of growth in body size. Table 9.2 summarises the results from multiple linear

TABLE 9.1

Summary Statistics of Body Weight Measurements (in kilograms, kg) and Blood Pressure (in millimetres of mercury) for 834 Girls in Cebu Cohort

			Pearson Correlations						
Variable	Mean	SD	$Weight_0$	$Weight_1$	$Weight_2$	$Weight_8$	$Weight_{15}$	$Weight_{19}$	SBP
$Weight_0$	2.96	0.42	1						
$Weight_1$	7.65	0.94	0.42	1					
$Weight_2$	9.45	1.08	0.42	0.82	1				
$Weight_8$	20.32	2.80	0.32	0.57	0.67	1			
$Weight_{15}$	41.90	6.31	0.31	0.46	0.51	0.76	1		
$Weight_{19}$	45.83	7.01	0.27	0.38	0.40	0.64	0.80	1	
SBP	99.32	9.20	−0.05	−0.01	−0.01	0.03	0.11	0.19	1

Note: $Weight_N$: N is the age at which body weight is measured. SD: standard deviation.

TABLE 9.2

Results from Multiple Linear Regression for *SBP* on Weight z-Scores at Different Ages

	Regression Coefficients	95% Confidence Intervals	t-Value	P-value
Intercept	96.11	90.03, 102.19	31.04	
zwt_0	−1.94	−3.55, −0.33	−2.36	0.018
zwt_1	−0.40	−1.55, 0.75	−0.68	0.496
zwt_2	0.36	−0.75, 1.46	0.63	0.527
zwt_8	−0.50	−0.89, −0.11	−2.52	0.012
zwt_{15}	0.01	−0.18, 0.20	0.09	0.926
zwt_{19}	0.40	0.25, 0.55	5.37	<0.001

regression analyses, and Figure 9.6 is the lifecourse plot for *SBP* regressed on the six body size z-scores (zwt_0, zwt_1, zwt_2, zwt_8, zwt_{15}, and zwt_{19}), between birth and age 19, in 834 girls. Regression coefficients in early life are all small, whereas those at 8 and 19 years are larger and of opposite sign, indicating that weight gain from 8 to 19 years (i.e., into and through puberty) is an important risk factor for high *SBP* at 19 years.

The potential difficulty in the interpretation of the lifecourse plot is collinearity amongst the series of body size measurements (for a discussion of collinearity, see Chapter 5). As growth is a continuous process, body size measurements are generally correlated, and the shorter the age interval between two measurements, the greater the correlation (Table 9.1). In Table 9.2, when all six body size measurements are included in the multiple regression, zwt_0, zwt_1 and zwt_8 have negative associations with *SBP*, yet zwt_1 and zwt_8 have positive bivariate correlations with *SBP* in Table 9.1. If body size was measured at age 17 years in the Cebu cohort, it would be highly correlated with zwt_{15}, zwt_{19} and *SBP*, and moderately with other variables. The

TABLE 9.3

Results from Multiple Linear Regression for *SBP*
on Weight z-Scores At Birth and Five Incremental
Changes in Weight z-Scores

	Regression Coefficients	95% Confidence Intervals
Model 1		
zwt_0	0.65	−0.16, 1.46
zwt_{1-0}	1.46	0.63, 2.29
zwt_{2-1}	1.84	0.64, 3.04
zwt_{8-2}	1.45	0.58, 2.33
zwt_{15-8}	2.87	1.89, 3.84
zwt_{19-15}	2.81	1.78, 3.84
Model 2		
zwt_{1-0}	0.81	0.14, 1.49
zwt_{2-1}	1.19	−0.01, 2.39
zwt_{8-2}	0.80	−0.13, 1.74
zwt_{15-8}	2.22	1.12, 3.31
zwt_{19-15}	2.16	1.00, 3.32
zwt_{19}	0.65	−0.16, 1.46

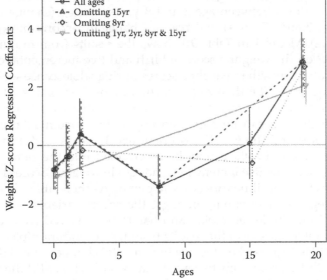

FIGURE 9.6
Lifecourse plot for *SBP* on weight z-scores during birth to age 19 years in 834 Cebu girls.

inclusion of body size at age 17 years in the lifecourse plot would substantially change the regression coefficients in the model and therefore change our interpretation of the plot. On the other hand, if one of the six body size measurements in the current plot is omitted, the new plot will look quite different. In Figure 9.6 we show the lifecourse plots for three alternative scenarios: (1) z-score weight at ages 15 years is omitted; (2) z-score weight at age 8 years is omitted; and (3) only z-score weights at birth and 19 years included. In scenario one, there is a large change in the regression coefficient between ages 15 and 19 years; in scenario two, the change is noted between ages 8 and 19 years. These results are not necessarily contradictory, as the body size measurements considered are sparse and there is no interim measurement between ages 8 and 19 years. However, since body sizes are correlated, and zwt_{19} has the largest correlation with SBP, the subtle effects of early postnatal growth may nevertheless be masked by collinearity.

9.2.2 Regression with Changes Scores

If our aim is to identify a critical period of time during the lifecourse in which rapid growth in body size is associated with an increased risk of chronic diseases in later life, an intuitive approach is to regress the disease outcome on the growth in body size in different periods of time during the lifecourse (Skidmore et al. 2007). In our example, there are six body weight z-scores during birth to age 19 years, so we may regress SBP on z-scores at birth (zwt_0) and five incremental changes in z-scores: zwt_{1-0} (change in z-scores between birth and age 1 year), zwt_{2-1} (change in z-scores between age 1 and 2 years), zwt_{8-2} (change in z-scores between age 2 and 8 years), zwt_{15-8} (change in z-scores between age 8 and 15 years), and zwt_{19-15} (change in z-scores between age 15 and 19 years). Model 1 in Table 9.3 shows the results from multiple regression for SBP on the weight z-score at birth and five incremental changes in weight z-scores. Growth in weight z-scores during adolescence seems to have a greater impact on SBP than early growth and birth size. It is interesting to note that the z-score weight at birth (zwt_0) has a positive association with SBP.

Alternatively, SBP can be regressed on the five incremental changes in weight z-scores and the weight z-score at age 19 years (zwt_{19}) instead. The reason that zwt_0 and zwt_{19} cannot be entertained into the same regression model along with the five incremental changes in weight z-scores is the problem of perfect multicollinearity (see Chapter 6). As there are only six dimensions (or degrees of freedom) amongst the seven variables, one becomes redundant in multiple regression and has to be removed from the model. Model 2 in Table 9.3 shows the results from the second multiple regression, in which SBP is regressed on the five incremental changes in weight z-scores and zwt_{19}. Whilst zwt_{19} seems to have the largest effect on SBP, the regression coefficients for the five incremental changes in weight z-scores in Model 2 have become much smaller than in Model 1, but later growth still has a larger effect than early growth. The question is, which set of regression coefficients for the five incremental changes—in Model 1 or Model 2—are to be inter-preted as the correct effects of the five incremental changes on *SBP*?

In fact, although those two sets of regression coefficient may look quite different, there is a simple mathematical relationship between them: for the same variables, regression coefficients in Model 1 = 0.65 + regression coeffi-cients in Model 2. To explain this simple mathematical relationship, however, requires some advanced mathematics, and we postpone the explanation to the next chapter on partial least-squares regression.

9.2.3 Latent Growth Curve Models

Latent growth curve models (LGCM) are a special type of structural equa-tion model for longitudinal data analysis. In Chapter 4 we used it to esti-mate the relation between changes and initial values, and we said, from a statistical viewpoint, that it is equivalent to multilevel modelling for longi-tudinal data analysis. However, LGCM is superior to multilevel models for analysing data from certain study designs, especially where incorporating latent variables into the model-building process is required. Book-length dis-cussions of LGCM can be found in Bollen and Curran (2006) and Duncan et al. (2006).

In multilevel models of longitudinal data, repeated measurements form level one, clustered within subjects at level two. For instance, the six body weights measured between birth and age 19 years are level-one variables clustered with the 960 boys in the Cebu cohort. A basic multilevel model would be a linear growth model; that is, a straight line is fitted to the six body weight measurements for each boy, yielding 960 straight lines (usually called *growth curves*), each with a different intercept and slope if fitted within the multilevel model with both random intercept and random slope (Hox 2002; Twisk 2006; Tu et al. 2009a). The distributions of the intercepts and slopes are assumed to follow a normal distribution, and their means and variances are estimated by minimising the differences between the observed and fitted values. The means of the fitted intercepts and slopes are called *fixed effects*, and their variances are called random effects. In contrast, the fitted inter-cepts and slopes of growth curves are explicitly modelled as latent variables in LGCM. Therefore, from the perspective of LGCM, the two-level multilevel model is a single-level model (Figure 9.7). The fixed and random effects in the multilevel models are estimated as the means and variances of the latent variables in LGCM (Bollen and Curran 2006; Tu et al. 2009a).

For the basic linear growth curve model, the two-level multilevel model for the 834 girls in the Cebu cohort is given as

$$Weight_{ij} = b_{0j}1 + b_{1j}Age_{ij} + e_{ij},\qquad(9.1)$$

where *Weight* and *Age* are recorded at the time each repeated measurement is taken; **1** is the identity vector (with values of one throughout); $b_{0j} = \beta_0 + u_{0j}$

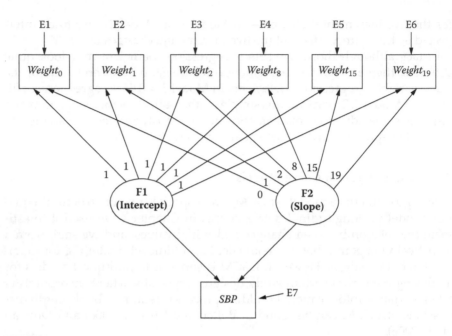

FIGURE 9.7
Path diagram for the linear latent growth curve model.

and $b_{1j} = \beta_1 + u_{1j}$ are, respectively, the random intercept and random slope with means β_0 and β_1 and variation given by

$$\begin{pmatrix} u_{0j} \\ u_{1j} \end{pmatrix} \sim N\left[\begin{pmatrix} 0 \\ 0 \end{pmatrix}, \begin{pmatrix} \sigma_{u0}^2 & \sigma_{u01} \\ \sigma_{u01} & \sigma_{u1}^2 \end{pmatrix} \right]$$

with variances σ_{u0}^2 and σ_{u1}^2; yielding a covariance σ_{u01}, $e_{ij} \sim N(0,\sigma_{e0}^2)$ as the residual error term, and $i = 1 \dots 6, j = 1 \dots 834$. Equation 9.1 can also be expressed as

$$Weight_{ij} = b_{0j} * \begin{bmatrix} 1 \\ 1 \\ 1 \\ 1 \\ 1 \\ 1 \end{bmatrix} + b_{1j} * \begin{bmatrix} 0 \\ 1 \\ 2 \\ 8 \\ 15 \\ 19 \end{bmatrix} + e_{ij}, \tag{9.2}$$

where it becomes clear that b_{0j} is the estimated birth weight and b_{1j} is the estimated gain in body weight in kilograms per year.

Equation 9.2 can be viewed as a combination of six single-level equations:

$$Weight_{1j} = b_{0j} * 1 + b_{1j} * 0 + e_{1j} , \qquad (9.3)$$

$$Weight_{2j} = b_{0j} * 1 + b_{1j} * 1 + e_{2j} , \qquad (9.4)$$

$$Weight_{3j} = b_{0j} * 1 + b_{1j} * 2 + e_{3j} , \qquad (9.5)$$

$$Weight_{4j} = b_{0j} * 1 + b_{1j} * 8 + e_{4j} , \qquad (9.6)$$

$$Weight_{5j} = b_{0j} * 1 + b_{1j} * 15 + e_{5j} , \qquad (9.7)$$

$$Weight_{6j} = b_{0j} * 1 + b_{1j} * 19 + e_{6j} , \qquad (9.8)$$

where $Weight_{1j}$ to $Weight_{6j}$ are body weights measured on occasion 1 (age 0; that is, at birth), 2 (age 1 year), 3 (age 2 years), 4 (age 8 years), 5 (age 15 years) and 6 (age 19 years). In multilevel models, b_{0j} and b_{1j} are regression coefficients with both fixed (β_0 and β_1) and random effects (σ_{u0}^2 and σ_{u1}^2); in LGCM, b_{0j} and b_{1j} are latent variables (denoted F1 and F2 in Figure 9.7), and their means and variances are estimated accordingly. The vector **1** and Age_{ij} are covariates in multilevel models (although the vector **1** for the intercept is not explicitly specified in most statistical software packages); in contrast, these two variables are specified as factor loadings for the relationships between the latent variables and their six indicator variables (i.e., the six body weight measurements) in LGCM. Therefore, in multilevel models, the longitudinal data is in the 'long' format; that is, the six body weights between birth and age 19 years are treated as repeated measurements and *stacked* in one column, whereas in LGCM, the six body weights are in the wide format; that is, treated as six different variables represented in matrix form as *adjacent* separate variables (not a single *stacked* variable).

In Figure 9.7, the factor loadings for the six body weights on F1 are all unity and, as a result, F1 becomes the estimated baseline body weight; that is, the estimated birth weights or "true" birth weight if we consider e_{1j} to be measurement errors in the observed birth weight. If the factor loadings for the six body weights on F2 are specified by following the chronological ages at which those weights were measured, F2 is interpreted as the estimated growth in weight per year since birth to age 19 years. The residual error terms e_{2j} to e_{6j} are the differences between estimated and observed body weights, so F2 is the estimated or true growth in weight, taking into account measurement errors.

Within lifecourse research, one important advantage of using the LGCM approach instead of multilevel models for estimating growth curves is that it is quite straightforward to test the effects of F1 and F2 on *SBP* in LGCM, as shown in Figure 9.7, because both the estimated intercepts and slopes in multilevel models are explicitly specified as latent variables in the LGCM model. Table 9.3 shows the results from the LGCM in Figure 9.7, and the effects of

TABLE 9.3

Results from Latent Growth Curve Models

			Linear Growth Curve Model						Nonlinear Growth Curve Model		
			Estimate	S.E.	P-value				Estimate	S.E.	P-value
Regression Weights											
$Weight_0$	←	F1	1			$Weight_0$	←	F1	1		
$Weight_1$	←	F1	1			$Weight_1$	←	F1	1		
$Weight_2$	←	F1	1			$Weight_2$	←	F1	1		
$Weight_8$	←	F1	1			$Weight_8$	←	F1	1		
$Weight_{15}$	←	F1	1			$Weight_{15}$	←	F1	1		
$Weight_{19}$	←	F1	1			$Weight_{19}$	←	F1	1		
$Weight_0$	←	F2	0			$Weight_0$	←	F2	0		
$Weight_1$	←	F2	1			$Weight_1$	←	F2	2.072	0.013	<0.001
$Weight_2$	←	F2	2			$Weight_2$	←	F2	2.867	0.015	<0.001
$Weight_8$	←	F2	8			$Weight_8$	←	F2	7.702	0.036	<0.001
$Weight_{15}$	←	F2	15			$Weight_{15}$	←	F2	17.283	0.083	<0.001
$Weight_{19}$	←	F2	19			$Weight_{19}$	←	F2	19		
SBP	←	F2	6.981	1.348	<0.001	SBP	←	F2	5.576	1.441	<0.001
SBP	←	F1	–1.721	0.506	<0.001	SBP	←	F1	–5.156	1.536	<0.001
Means											
F1			5.253	0.031	<0.001	F1			2.966	0.015	<0.001
F2			2.145	0.012	<0.001	F2			2.256	0.013	<0.001
Covariances											
F1	↔	F2	0.007	0.011	0.527	F1	↔	F2	0.028	0.005	0.045
Variances											
F1			0.570	0.040	<0.001	F1			0.103	0.011	<0.001
F2			0.083	0.006	<0.001	F2			0.077	0.004	<0.001
E1			5.775	0.290	<0.001	E1			0.086	0.011	<0.001
E2			0.287	0.025	<0.001	E2			0.382	0.022	<0.001
E3			0.240	0.024	<0.001	E3			0.445	0.027	<0.001
E4			21.993	1.148	<0.001	E4			1.999	0.133	<0.001
E5			35.621	1.978	<0.001	E5			12.072	0.762	<0.001
E6			15.595	1.486	<0.001	E6			21.081	1.221	<0.001
E7			78.904	4.057	<0.001	E7			80.92	4.124	<0.001

Note: S.E.: standard errors.

F1 (birth weight) and F2 (growth in weight) on *SBP* are –1.72 mmHg/kg and 6.98 mmHg/kg, respectively, suggesting that there is an inverse relationship between *SBP* and birth weight and a positive association between *SBP* and current weight.

However, this model has a very large chi-squared value (6212, degrees of freedom [DF] = 20), indicating a poor model fit. This is not surprising, as Figure 9.5 clearly indicates that the growth in body weight does not follow a linear pattern. There are many ways of specifying and estimating nonlinear growth curves, such as estimating quadratic or cubic curves in multilevel models, but LGCM provides a simple and elegant approach to estimating nonlinear growth by freeing the factor loadings of the middle four body weights on F2. If the growth pattern was indeed linear, the estimated factor loadings would be close to those previously specified; that is, 1, 2, 8 and 15, respectively. Table 9.3 shows the results of the nonlinear model where the four factor loadings are estimated to be 2.07, 2.87, 7.70 and 17.28, respectively. This indicates that the growth *speed* between birth and year 1 is about twice as fast as that on average for the remaining period. The speed of weight gain is faster again between the ages 8 and 15 years, and slows after the age of 15 years. In the nonlinear model, the effects of F1 (birth weight) and F2 (growth in weight) on *SBP* are –5.16 mmHg/kg and 5.58 mmHg/kg, respectively. The model chi-squared value has reduced to 854.6 (DF = 16).

In a review article on statistical issues in lifecourse epidemiology, De Stavola and her colleagues (2006) proposed the use of LGCM to estimate the effects of growth throughout different periods of lifecourse on later-life health outcomes. The basic idea is to take advantage of the flexibility of LGCM in estimating growth in body size during different periods of the lifecourse. For instance, suppose we would like to estimate the effect of early (between birth and age 8) and later (between age 8 to 19) growth in body weight on *SBP*. We could set up three latent variables in the two-phase latent growth curve model: F1 is the intercept, F2 is the growth in body weight between birth and age 2, and F3 is the growth between age 2 to age 19 (Figure 9.8). Factor loadings of the body weights on F1 are fixed to unity, as they were in Figure 9.7; factor loadings of the six body weights on F2 are fixed to 0, 1, 2, 2, 2 and 2; and the factor loadings of the six body weights on F3 are fixed to 0, 0, 0, 6, 13 and 17. From a multilevel modelling perspective, this latent growth model with three latent variables is a spline model (Fitzmaurice et al. 2004):

$$Weight_{ij} = b_{0j} * \begin{bmatrix} 1 \\ 1 \\ 1 \\ 1 \\ 1 \\ 1 \end{bmatrix} + b_{1j} * \begin{bmatrix} 0 \\ 1 \\ 2 \\ 2 \\ 2 \\ 2 \end{bmatrix} + b_{2j} * \begin{bmatrix} 0 \\ 0 \\ 0 \\ 6 \\ 13 \\ 17 \end{bmatrix} + e_{ij}, \tag{9.9}$$

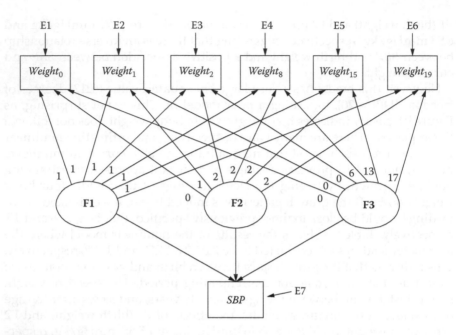

FIGURE 9.8
Path diagram for the two-phase linear latent growth curve model. To simplify the presentation, the covariances between latent variances F1 to F3 are omitted.

where $b_{0j} = \beta_0 + u_{0j}$, $b_{1j} = \beta_1 + u_{1j}$ and $b_{2j} = \beta_2 + u_{2j}$ are, respectively, the random intercept and random slopes with means β_0, β_1 and β_2 with random variation described by

$$
\begin{pmatrix} u_{0j} \\ u_{1j} \\ u_{2j} \end{pmatrix} \sim N \left[\begin{pmatrix} 0 \\ 0 \\ 0 \end{pmatrix}, \begin{pmatrix} \sigma_{u0}^2 & \sigma_{u01} & \sigma_{u02} \\ \sigma_{u01} & \sigma_{u1}^2 & \sigma_{u12} \\ \sigma_{u02} & \sigma_{u12} & \sigma_{u2}^2 \end{pmatrix} \right]
$$

with variances σ_{u0}^2, σ_{u1}^2 and σ_{u2}^2, yielding three covariances σ_{u01}, σ_{u02} and σ_{u12}.
Note that the sum of the two vectors is equal to the chronological age:

$$
\begin{bmatrix} 0 \\ 1 \\ 2 \\ 2 \\ 2 \\ 2 \end{bmatrix} + \begin{bmatrix} 0 \\ 0 \\ 0 \\ 6 \\ 13 \\ 17 \end{bmatrix} = \begin{bmatrix} 0 \\ 1 \\ 2 \\ 8 \\ 15 \\ 19 \end{bmatrix}.
$$

The difference between this model and the previous one is that this model estimates different linear weight gain velocities between birth and age 2, and between age 2 and 19. For example, at age 15, the estimated weight is b_0 (estimated average birth weight) + b_1 * 2 (estimated weight gain per year between birth and age 2 times two) + b_2 * 13 (estimated weight gain per year between age 2 and age 19 times 13). Although different growth curve velocities are estimated for the two phases of the lifecourse, the velocity in body weight gain is still assumed to be constant within each phase. Results from the nonlinear model (Table 9.3), however, have already indicated that the assumption of linear growth within these two phases may not be correct, and indeed the LGCM with three latent variables has a very poor fit and has two negative residual variances. As variances should always be positive values, this indicates that the model has been mis-specified.

Equation 9.9 can also be viewed as a combination of six single-level equations:

$$Weight_{1j} = b_{0j} * 1 + b_{1j} * 0 + b_{2j} * 0 + e_{1j}, \tag{9.10}$$

$$Weight_{2j} = b_{0j} * 1 + b_{1j} * 1 + b_{2j} * 0 + e_{2j}, \tag{9.11}$$

$$Weight_{3j} = b_{0j} * 1 + b_{1j} * 2 + b_{2j} * 0 + e_{3j}, \tag{9.12}$$

$$Weight_{4j} = b_{0j} * 1 + b_{1j} * 2 + b_{2j} * 6 + e_{4j}, \tag{9.13}$$

$$Weight_{5j} = b_{0j} * 1 + b_{1j} * 2 + b_{2j} * 13 + e_{5j}, \tag{9.14}$$

$$Weight_{6j} = b_{0j} * 1 + b_{1j} * 2 + b_{2j} * 15 + e_{6j}, \tag{9.15}$$

In LGCM, the variation in estimated intercept and slopes are treated as three latent variables, their means are the fixed effects in Equation 9.10, and their variances and covariances are the random effects.

To accommodate nonlinear growth in the two phases of growth in body weight, we free the factor loading of $Weight_1$ on F2, and the factor loadings of $Weight_8$ and $Weight_{15}$ on F3 in the two-phase model; that is, we no longer assume that the growth velocity is constant between birth and age 2 or between age 2 and age 19. These modifications greatly improve the model fit (chi-squared = 84.6, DF = 12, $P < 0.001$; Root-Mean-Square Error of Approximation (RMSEA) = 0.085; Comparative Fix Index (CFI) = 0.978). The factor loading of $Weight_1$ on F2 is 1.44, indicating that growth in weight is greater in the first than the second year (Table 9.4). The factor loadings of $Weight_8$ and $Weight_{15}$ are 5.08 and 15.20, respectively, indicating that the growth velocity in weight between ages 8 and 15 is greater than both that between ages 2 and 8 and that between ages 15 and 19. The average weight gain during the first 2 years since birth is 3.24 kg per year, and the average weight gain between ages 2 and 19 is 2.14 kg per year. However, whilst gain in body weight between ages 2 and 19 has a positive effect on *SBP*, the effect

TABLE 9.4

Results from the Two-Phase Latent Growth
Curve Model

			Estimate	S.E.	P-value
Regression Weights					
$Weight_0$	←	F1	1		
$Weight_1$	←	F1	1		
$Weight_2$	←	F1	1		
$Weight_8$	←	F1	1		
$Weight_{15}$	←	F1	1		
$Weight_{19}$	←	F1	1		
$Weight_0$	←	F2	0		
$Weight_1$	←	F2	1.443	0.006	<0.001
$Weight_2$	←	F2	2		
$Weight_8$	←	F2	2		
$Weight_{15}$	←	F2	2		
$Weight_{19}$	←	F2	2		
$Weight_8$	←	F3	5.079	0.03	<0.001
$Weight_{15}$	←	F3	15.196	0.064	<0.001
$Weight_{19}$	←	F3	17		
SBP	←	F1	−3.591	1.635	0.028
SBP	←	F2	−0.372	0.881	0.672
SBP	←	F3	5.404	1.116	<0.001
Means					
F1			2.963	0.015	<0.001
F2			3.243	0.017	<0.001
F3			2.137	0.014	<0.001
Covariances					
F1	↔	F2	0.039	0.015	0.010
F2	↔	F3	0.053	0.006	<0.001
F1	↔	F3	0.04	0.005	<0.001
Variances					
F1			0.113	0.027	<0.001
F2			0.214	0.015	<0.001
F3			0.117	0.006	<0.001
E1			0.066	0.026	0.012
E2			0.258	0.017	<0.001
E3			0.041	0.021	0.049
E4			2.199	0.127	<0.001
E5			5.142	0.552	<0.001
E6			13.403	0.919	<0.001
E7			81.201	4.045	<0.001

of weight gain between birth and age 2 is small and negative; birth weight has a negative effect on *SBP*.

Using LGCM to estimate the effects of growth in the lifecourse is more flexible than multiple regression as it is straightforward to incorporate latent variables into the model. However, the number of latent variables for the different phases of the lifecourse in the growth model is limited by the number of body size measurements. When more latent variables are included in the model to estimate the effects of growth in different phases of the lifecourse, the number of parameters such as means, variances and covariances will increase substantially. This can cause problems with model identification, giving rise to nonconvergence in the estimation process, or the model may converge to unacceptable results, for example, some variances are negative.

Another contentious issue is that how the phases are demarcated is more or less arbitrary. In our example, we assume that the growth between birth and age 2 has a different impact from the growth between ages 2 to 19. This demarcation is partly due to when the body weights were measured, but there are still several other options. If we divide the two phases using age 8, we will get different results, and we are not able to estimate the effect between birth and age 2 on *SBP*. On the other hand, if body size is intensively measured throughout the lifecourse (e.g., every 6 months), it becomes quite challenging to define which growth phases during the lifecourse should be adopted by the LGCM approach. Another, and probably the most serious, limitation is that the use of LGCM currently requires that the measurements of body size are more or less made at the same ages for the entire cohort. Otherwise, setting up the latent variables correctly could become quite tedious and the model may not be identifiable.

In our illustration of the lifecourse plot, we used weight z-scores, but in LGCM we use the original body weights. This is because the mean values of the six weight z-scores are all zero by definition. Therefore, from the perspective of the whole population, there is no change in the means of weight z-scores; that is, there is no 'growth' in weights. However, technically, it is still possible to use weight z-scores in LGCM to test the effects of growth in different phases of the lifecourse, though the results and their interpretation will be different. For raw weight scores, the interpretation is the effect of weight change in 1 kg, but for weight z-scores, it is the effect of change in the rank of weight in the sample/population. Which one (raw weights or z-score weights) should be used depends upon the biological theory. For example, if we are interested in the effect of weight gain in early childhood, raw weight scores seems to be the more sensible choice. However, if we are interested in the effect of catch-up growth, weight z-scores seem to provide a better approach.

9.2.4 Growth Mixture Models

In the social sciences, two recently developed methods have been used to identify trajectories for subgroups. Group-based modelling has been widely used in criminology to identify the trajectory in delinquency for repeated offenders in adulthood (Nagin 1999, 2001, 2005). Growth mixture modelling (Muthén and Muthén 2000) is an extension of latent growth curve modelling and has been widely used in developmental psychology. Although there are differences in the philosophical thinking behind these two methods, they can be considered statistically related (Kreuter and Muthén 2008). As explained in the Section 9.2.3, traditional linear mixed modelling for longitudinal data estimates individual growth trajectories, and the variations in model intercepts and slopes (i.e., the random effects) are assumed to follow a normal distribution (Goldstein 1995; Hox 2002). The random effects in linear mixed models can be seen as latent continuous variables and are actually modelled as latent variables in latent growth curve modelling (Bollen and Curran 2006). In both group-based modelling and growth mixture modelling, the latent variables capturing the random effects are modelled as categorical variables; that is, latent classes. In group-based modelling, whilst different classes have different growth trajectories, subjects within each class are assumed to have identical intercepts (i.e., baseline values) and slopes (i.e., trajectories); that is, no within-class variation is assumed in the estimation of class memberships (Nagin 1999, 2005). In contrast, whilst the random effects are modelled as categorical variables in growth mixture modelling, within-class variations are allowed in the estimation of class memberships; that is, within each class the random effects are modelled as continuous variables (Kreuter and Muthén 2008). Therefore, conceptually, group-based modelling can be considered a special case of growth mixture modelling where all within-class variations are constrained to be zero.

To illustrate growth mixture modelling, we uses the macro PROC TRAJ (Jones et al. 2001) for the statistical software SAS® (version 9.1.3) to analyse the body weight z-scores from birth to age 19 in the 960 boys in the Cebu cohort. To capture the subtle features in growth trajectories, we fit a quartic curve for each group. We start with the two-class model and gradually increase the number of classes.

Figure 9.9 illustrates the concepts behind the group-based model using a path diagram. Latent variable C in Figure 9.9 represents the classes, and the arrows from C to each of the growth curve parameters (intercepts, linear slopes, quadratic, cubic and quartic) indicate that these parameters are different across the classes; that is, each class has its own distinct average growth trajectory. However, in group-based modelling, it is assumed that there is no within-group variation; that is, the variances of the five latent variables F1 to F5 are constrained to be zero. Figure 9.10 shows the growth curves for each latent class in different models. In the two-class model, class-1 comprises men who were born smaller and who remained slightly smaller, whilst class-2 comprises men who were born larger and remained slightly larger. The average *SBP* values in class-1 and class-2 are 98.85 and 99.90 mmHg, respectively, and this difference is not statistically significant (1.05 mmHg, 95% CI = −0.21,

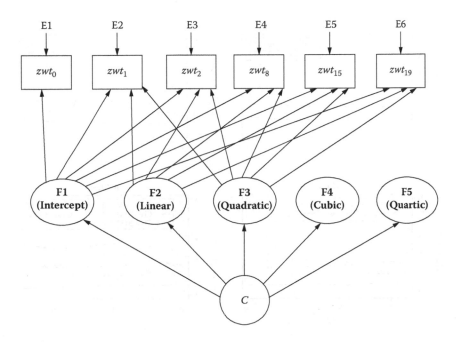

FIGURE 9.9
Path diagram for group-based models. To simplify the presentation, the arrows from F4 and F5 to the six body weights are omitted.

2.30). In the three-class model, the first two classes are similar to the two classes in the two-class model. The additional third class comprises women who were born larger than average and become much larger after the age of 8 years. About 18% of women are in this class. The average *SBP* values in class 1, class 2 and class 3 are 98.5, 99.4 and 100.6 mmHg, respectively, and the contrast between class 1 and class 3 is statistically significant (2.13 mmHg, 95%CI: 0.30, 3.96).

In the four-class model, the differences between the first three classes are small compared to the differences between each of these classes and class-4 (Figure 9.10 and Table 9.5). The increase in body weight z-scores since birth in class-4 is more striking than that in class-3 for the 3-class model. However, only 73 young women (8.6%) are in this extreme class. Class 4 has the highest *SBP*, and the difference in mean *SBP* between class-1 and class 4 was statistically significant.

In the five-class model, class 3 is similar to class 4 in the four-class model and has the highest *SBP* (Figure 9.10 and Table 9.5). However, it is noted that class-5, which comprises women who were born large and remained relatively large, did not have greater *SBP* compared to those who were born small and remained small (e.g., class 1).

In our illustration, we use weight z-scores for growth mixture modelling, though we can also use original weight measurements. Since body

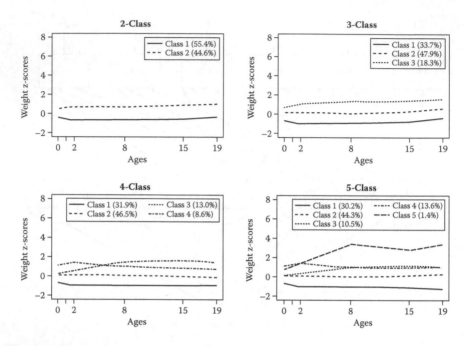

FIGURE 9.10
Growth trajectories identified by group-based models with different numbers of classes.

weights in general increase with age (see Figure 9.5), the trajectories of original weights will look quite different from those for weight z-scores during the early lifecourse period.

9.3 Discussion

In this chapter we use data from the Cebu cohort to illustrate different approaches to testing the relationship between growth in body size throughout the lifecourse and blood pressure. Each approach has its advantages and limitations. Tracing the lifecourse body size z-scores of subjects with chronic diseases in later life seems straightforward and informative. However, the apparent associations between growth trajectories and adverse adult health outcomes manifest from the changes in the magnitude of *cross-sectional* relationships between body size and adult health outcomes with increasing age. The observed association of growth patterns, such as those in Figures 9.1 and 9.4, with adverse health outcomes in later life only confirm what is already known—that adult body sizes have a positive relationship with later-life adverse health outcomes, and body sizes at birth or during early childhood have weaker, inverse relationships.

TABLE 9.5

Average *SBP* in Each Class in Different Group-Based Models

	Mean	S.D.	No. of Subjects	Difference[a]	95% CI	P-value
2-Class Model (BIC = –6,416.53, AIC = –6,388.17)						
Class-1	98.85	9.57	460			
Class-2	99.90	8.69	374	1.05	(–0.21, 2.30)	0.10
3-Class Model (BIC = –6,214.37, AIC = –6,171.83)						
Class-1	98.49	9.72	278			
Class-2	99.41	8.78	407	0.92	(–0.48, 2.33)	0.196
Class-3	100.62	9.20	149	2.13	(0.30, 3.96)	0.022
4-Class Model (BIC= –6,112.31, AIC= –6,055.59)						
Class-1	98.33	9.76	262			
Class-2	99.60	8.73	401	1.26	(–0.16, 2.69)	0.082
Class-3	98.87	9.22	98	0.54	(–1.59, 2.66)	0.622
Class-4	101.98	9.11	73	3.65	(1.27, 6.03)	0.003
5-Class Model (BIC = –6,069.67, AIC = –5,998.78)						
Class-1	98.24	9.78	250			
Class-2	99.50	8.77	380	1.26	(–0.20, 2.73)	0.090
Class-3	102.16	8.49	85	3.93	(1.67, 6.18)	0.001
Class-4	99.10	9.08	108	0.86	(–1.21, 2.93)	0.416
Class-5	98.00	12.50	11	–0.24	(–5.77, 5.29)	0.933

[a] The reference class is Class-1 in each model.

Some studies have found greater associations between catch-up growth trajectories and later-life health outcomes in one sex more than the other (Barker et al. 2005). However, this simply indicates that the associations between body sizes at each age and later-life health outcomes are different for men and women.

The lifecourse plot is also a simple approach, but collinearity amongst body sizes can make the interpretation of the plot quite challenging. Latent growth curve modelling seems to provide a more flexible framework for estimating the effects of growth velocity in different phases of the lifecourse. Nevertheless, as shown, patterns of growth trajectories need to be correctly specified, and there is usually more than one choice of dividing the lifecourse into different phases, which can yield multiple model parameterisations that could be interpreted differently. Moreover, using latent growth curve modelling usually requires that the measurements are undertaken at the same ages for the whole cohort, which is rarely stringently satisfied.

Growth mixture modelling is a recent development and extension of latent growth curve modelling, and it seems to provide a sophisticated approach to identifying distinctive growth trajectories in the population. However, model specifications are again sometimes arbitrary and the selection of the optimal model is not always straightforward. For instance, Akaike Information Criterion (AIC) and Bayesian Information Criterion (BIC) values have been used for selecting the optimal number of classes in a group-based model (Nagin 2005; Bollen and Curran 2006):

$$\text{AIC} = -2\log(L) + 2k, \tag{9.16}$$

and

$$\text{BIC} = -2\log(L) + k * \log(N), \tag{9.17}$$

where L is the value of the model's maximised likelihood, N is the sample size and k the number of free parameters in the model. Both indices can be viewed as a penalised model-fit index by taking into account the number of free parameters (the more complex the model, the greater the number of free parameter) and sample size. The smaller the AIC or BIC, the more parsimonious the model is. Note that some statistical software packages used slightly different formula, so AIC and BIC have negative values (e.g., multiplying Equation 9.16 and 9.17 by −0.5). Therefore, the greater the AIC or BIC, the more parsimonious the model is. This is what PROC TRAJ actually does.

In our example of the 834 girls in the Cebu cohort, the 5-class model has the largest AIC and BIC values, but the AIC and BIC become even larger in the 6-class and 7-class models. However, whilst the latter might have a larger AIC or BIC, the additional classes are not easy to interpret, as the differences in the features in the trajectories amongst most classes also become much smaller. Furthermore, in our analysis, there is no within-class variation for the estimated growth curves, but if we allow the estimation of variances for the latent variables such as F1 and F2 in Figure 9.9, using, say, the software package Mplus, the growth trajectories might look quite different. For this reason, model selection for any lifecourse growth model must be driven as much by model interpretation as by likelihood-based model-fit criteria (Gilthorpe et al. 2009). Another practical issue is estimation problems in mixture models. As mixture models such as group-based modelling or growth mixture modelling usually entail complex likelihood functions, algorithms may converge to local minima/maxima that may lead to erroneous conclusions (Bauer 2007). Also, if the growth model is too complex, the algorithms may never converge when the number of classes and sample size are large, as the computations become so slow. On the other hand, if we only choose simple growth models for each class, the results may not be trustworthy. For example, longitudinal data usually require specification of complex autocorrelation structure amongst repeated measurements. Misspecification of correlation structure may give rise to biased estimation of the fixed effects. This specific issue is discussed in detail elsewhere (Gilthorpe et al. submitted). In the next chapter we will discuss how to use the partial least-squares technique to overcome some of the limitations of these current approaches.

10

Partial Least Squares Regression
for Lifecourse Research

10.1 Introduction

In Chapter 9, we discussed several approaches to identifying growth patterns/trajectories and estimating the effects of growth in different phases of the lifecourse on health in later life. One problem amongst many others is the collinearity between body size measurements during the lifecourse, which may cause unstable regression coefficients (see Chapter 6). Another problem is regression to the mean, such as that in tracing the mean z-scores for subjects with chronic diseases in later life.

One statistical challenge in lifecourse research is to distinguish the effects of birth size, growth in body size, and current body size (Lucas et al. 1999; Tu et al. 2006a, 2007). When there are only measurements of birth size and current body size (hence growth is known also), it is not feasible to estimate the *independent* contributions of the three variables conditional on the other two using ordinary least squares (OLS) multiple regression. This is because growth in body size, defined as the difference in current body size from birth size, yields perfect collinearity amongst the three variables, such that only two of the three variables can be entered into OLS regression; and this is regardless of which pair of variables is used, since mathematical relationships exist between pairs of regression coefficients in different models. Moreover, interpretation of the conditional relationships in OLS regression remains controversial, as a small negative association between birth size and later-life health outcome usually becomes much larger after the adjustment of current body size (see Chapter 7).

The problem of perfect collinearity in distinguishing the effects of birth size, growth in body size at different phases of the lifecourse, and current body size will not be overcome by increasing the number of body size measurements throughout the lifecourse even though this provides greater information on growth during the lifecourse. In this chapter we explain and illustrate an alternative approach to estimating the effects on later-life health outcomes of body size at different stages of the lifecourse using partial least squares (PLS) regression (Phatak et al. 1992; de Jong 1993; Phatak and de Jong 1997; Wold et al. 2001). PLS was developed in the 1970s and 1980s, and since has been widely used in chemometrics to overcome estimation problems in OLS regression, such as with highly collinear covariates and where the number of covariates exceed the number of independent observations. Whilst PLS has become a popular tool for data analysis in bioinformatics (Boulestrix and Strimmer 2007; Hastie et al. 2009), it has been rarely used in medical statistics and epidemiology. In this chapter we again use data from the Cebu birth cohort (see Chapter 9 for the details) to explain why PLS regression can overcome the problem of perfect collinearity in OLS regression and demonstrate how PLS may be used to estimate the effects of multiple body sizes throughout the lifecourse on later-life health outcomes. As PLS is rarely used in epidemiology, we will compare its results to those from OLS regression.

10.2 Data

In this chapter we again use postnatal data of body weights measured immediately after birth, aged 1 year, 2 years, 8 years, 15 years and 19 years from the Cebu cohort as we did in Chapter 9. The later-life health outcome is average systolic blood pressure (SBP) measured at age 19 years. In our demonstration we use data on the 834 girls without any missing measurements of body weight or blood pressure. Growth in body weight is defined as the change in weight z-scores between consecutive measurements; for example, growth in body weight between birth and age 1 ($zwt_{1-0} = zwt_1 - zwt_0$) is the difference in weight z-scores between birth (zwt_0) and age at 1 year (zwt_1). Note that if growth in body weight was defined as the change in raw body weight, we might get different results. Therefore, the change in weight z-scores is better interpreted as change in the relative body size in the sample population. A summary of the data has been shown already in Table 9.1 in Chapter 9.

10.3 OLS Regression

We first regress SBP on z-score birth weight (zwt_0), z-score current weight (zwt_{19}), and changes in weight z-scores between birth and age 19 (z_{19-0}), both separately and in pairs, as this is the most commonly reported analysis in the literature (see Chapter 6 for a discussion of the problems with this approach). SBP is then regressed on zwt_0, changes in weight z-scores between birth and age 1 (zwt_{1-0}), changes in weight z-scores between ages 1 and 2

(zwt_{2-1}), changes in weight z-scores between ages 2 and 8 (zwt_{8-2}), changes in weight z-scores between ages 8 and 15 (zwt_{15-8}), and changes in weight z-scores between ages 15 and 19 (zwt_{19-15}). In a separate analysis, *SBP* and diastolic blood pressure (DBP) are regressed simultaneously on the five successive weight z-score increments and the final weight z-score.

Table 10.1 shows that, within univariable regression models, zwt_0 had a small, non-significant inverse association with *SBP* (–0.48 mmHg/kg, 95% CI = –1.10, 0.14); and both zwt_{19-0} and zwt_{19} had a significantly positive association with *SBP* (zwt_{19-0}: 1.52, 95% CI = 1.02, 2.03; and zwt_{19}: 1.79, 95% CI = 1.14, 2.36). Within multivariable regression models, zwt_0 had a larger inverse association with *SBP* when zwt_{19} was adjusted for (–1.03, 95% CI = –1.65, –0.40), and had a positive association when zwt_{19-0} was adjusted for (2.03, 95% CI = 1.40, 2.66). Nevertheless, these two regression coefficients are of the same size in the opposite direction, depending upon whether zwt_{19} or zwt_{19-0} is adjusted for. We have discussed this phenomenon in Chapter 7.

Table 10.2 shows that when *SBP* is regressed on zwt_0 and the five successive weight z-scores increments simultaneously, all covariates have a positive association with the outcome, though the regression coefficient for zwt_0 is the smallest. When *SBP* is regressed on the five successive weight z-score increments and zwt_{19} simultaneously, the covariate zwt_{15-8} has the largest association with the outcome. The regression coefficient for zwt_{19} is *identical* to those for zwt_0 in the previous model (a similar finding is noted in Table 10.1). Figure 10.1 provides a graphical presentation of the regression coefficients for the two multivariable regression models in Table 10.2. If we ignore zwt_0 and zwt_{19} in the graphs, the two lines are actually parallel. We will give an explanation for this intriguing finding in the next section.

10.4 PLS Regression

10.4.1 History of PLS

The pioneering work of PLS was largely done by the distinguished Swedish econometrician and statistician Herman Wold in the 1960s and 1970s. In the 1960s, Herman Wold developed algorithms for solving eigenvalue problems for example, for principal component analysis and canonical correlation (Geladi 1988). His algorithms were called *non linear iterative partial least squares* (NIPALS). Wold had a PhD student in the 1960s working on factor analysis, and that student later became well known for his invaluable contributions to the development of maximum likelihood approach to structural equation modelling (SEM). The student was Karl Jöreskog. In the 1970s, Jöreskog proposed a unified theory for SEM based on maximum likelihood estimations, and his software Lisrel became almost the synonym for SEM. In view of the

TABLE 10.1

Results from the Univariable and Multivariable Linear Regression Models for 834 Girls

SBP	Univariable Regression		Multivariable Regression 1		Multivariable Regression 2		Multivariable Regression 3	
	Coefficient	95% CI	Coefficient	95% CI	Coefficient	95% CI	Coefficient	95% CI
zwt_0	−0.48	(−1.10, 0.14)	1.00	(0.24, 1.77)	−1.03	(−1.65, −0.40)		
zwt_{19-0}	1.52	(1.02, 2.03)	2.03	(1.40, 2.66)			1.03	(0.40, 1.65)
zwt_{19}	1.79	(1.14, 2.36)			2.03	(1.40, 2.66)	1.00	(0.24, 1.77)
R^2			4.8%		4.8%		4.8%	

Note: The outcome (systolic blood pressure [SBP]) regressed on each or two of the three body size measurements: z-score birth weight (zwt_0), z-score current body weight (zwt_{19}) and the difference in z-score between birth and current body weight (zwt_{19-0}).

TABLE 10.2

Results from the Univariable and Multivariable Linear Regression Models for 834 Girls

SBP	Univariable Regression		Multivariable Regression 1		Multivariable Regression 2	
	Coefficient	95% CI	Coefficient	95% CI	Coefficient	95% CI
zwt_0	−0.48	(−1.10, 0.14)	0.65	(−0.16, 1.46)		
zwt_{1-0}	0.33	(−0.24, 0.91)	1.46	(0.63, 2.29)	0.81	(0.14, 1.49)
zwt_{2-1}	0.14	(−0.91, 0.18)	1.84	(0.64, 3.04)	1.19	(−0.01, 2.40)
zwt_{8-2}	0.42	(−0.35, 1.20)	1.45	(0.58, 2.33)	0.80	(−0.13, 1.74)
zwt_{15-8}	1.67	(0.77, 2.56)	2.87	(1.89, 3.84)	2.22	(1.13, 3.31)
zwt_{19-15}	1.83	(0.84, 2.81)	2.81	(1.78, 3.84)	2.16	(1.00, 3.32)
zwt_{19}	1.79	(1.14, 2.36)			0.65	(−0.16, 1.46)
R^2			6.02%		6.02%	

Note: The results are for (1) the outcome *SBP* on each of the seven z-scores body weight or change in z-score weight, (2) on either z-score birth weight (zwt_0), the differences in z-score between birth and age 1 year (zwt_{1-0}), between age 1 year and 2 years (zwt_{2-1}), between age 2 years and 8 years (zwt_{8-2}), between age 8 years and 15 years (zwt_{15-8}), between age 15 years and 19 years (zwt_{19-15}), or (3) on zwt_{1-0}, zwt_{2-1}, zwt_{8-2}, zwt_{15-8}, zwt_{19-15} and z-score current body weight (zwt_{19}).

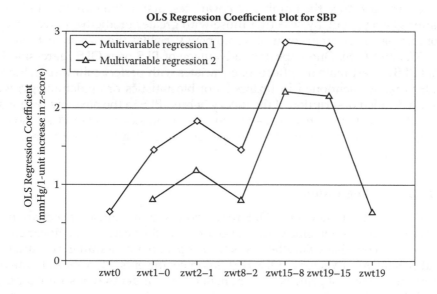

FIGURE 10.1

Graphical presentation of OLS regression coefficients for *SBP* regressed on six of the seven variables for birth weight z-score, five successive z-score weight increments and current body weight z-score.

success of the Lisrel approach to SEM, Wold felt that his NIPALS algorithms could also be used as an estimation method for path analysis, and he called his approach *soft modelling*, because, unlike the Lisrel approach, NIPAL does not require a full specification of the model, including the stochastic properties of residuals. For example, two important assumptions behind Lisrel or covariance-based SEM are multivariate normality and the independence of residuals. There is no such requirement for PLS path analysis, and this is why Wold called his PLS approach 'soft modelling' (Wold 1982), as it was devised as a method to explore multivariate relationships without strong theory or knowledge for guiding the model-building process. Later in the 1970s and 1980s, Herman Wold's son, Svente Wold, a chemist, saw the potential of PLS for dimension reduction for data with a limited number of observations but nevertheless with a large number of explanatory variables. Since then, PLS regression became an important tool for chemometricians, and major developments in PLS have been carried out by them. In bioinformatics, researchers encounter similar problems with data dimension reduction, and PLS regression has become an important analytical tool.

PLS regression gradually drew attention from statisticians, and in a seminal paper, Stone and Brooks (1990) showed that PLS can be viewed as an extension of principal component analysis (PCA). Along with PCA and OLS regression, PLS is a member of the family of continuum regression (Stone and Brooks 1990). Like PCA, PLS is also a data dimension reduction method; that is, when there are many collinear covariates in the model, it is sometimes necessary to reduce the number of covariates, due to the number of observations being small, by selecting those with greater predictive power or by combining the original covariates into new variables (known as *components* in PCA and PLS). One important advantage of PLS over OLS regression is that PLS can estimate the effects of covariates with perfect collinearity. Since PLS is rarely mentioned in textbooks of biostatistics or epidemiology, we give a detailed description of the theory behind PLS in the next few sections. Also, because PLS regression can be viewed as an extension of PCA regression, we start with a recap of PCA regression (see Chapter 6) and then move on to PLS.

10.4.2 PCA Regression

From a statistical viewpoint, OLS regression is to maximise the covariance between the $n \times 1$ outcome variable vector $\mathbf{y}$ and the vector of the linear combination of covariates $\mathbf{X\beta}$, where $\mathbf{X}$ is the $n \times p$ matrix containing p covariates and β is the $p \times 1$ vector of OLS regression coefficients. PCA seeks to maximise the variance of principal component $\mathbf{t}_1 = \mathbf{Xc}_1$ under the constraint for the modulus of the $p \times 1$ vector $\mathbf{c}_1$ to be unity. Successive principal components, $\mathbf{t}_2 = \mathbf{Xc}_2$, $\mathbf{t}_3 = \mathbf{Xc}_3$, etc., are obtained by repeating the procedure on the residuals from the preceding step, and all new principal components are uncorrelated with the preceding ones. The extraction of principal components is associated with a mathematical technique known, in matrix algebra, as singular value decomposition, which requires the calculation of eigenvectors and eigenvalues (Jackson 2003). For p variables, x_1, x_2, ..., x_p, each principal component, pc_i, is a weighted composite of p covariates:

$$pc_i = w_{i1}x_1 + w_{i2}x_2 + ... + w_{ip}x_p,$$ (10.1)

where w_{ij}, j = 1 to p, is the weight for covariate x_p in principal component pc_i. As we explained in Chapter 6 on collinearity, for six variables without perfect multicollinearity, six principal components, which are weighted combinations of the original six covariates, can be extracted. Note that in the construction of principal components, variables x_1, x_2, ..., x_p are usually in standardised form; that is, they have zero means and standard deviations equal to 1. The extracted principal components are ordered by the amount of total variance across the covariates that is explained by the components; that is, pc_1 explains more variance than pc_2, and pc_2 explains more than pc_3, etc. The first few principal components that explain most of the covariate variance are used as revised covariates for OLS regression. Note that if all six principal components were selected as covariates, the results from PCA regression, such as regression coefficients and R^2, would be equivalent to those from OLS regression. When the outcome is only regressed on the first few components, results will be different. One drawback in using PCA, as we explained in Chapter 6, is that the extraction of principal components does not take into account the relationship of the outcome with any of the covariates. In extreme cases, the discarded principal components might explain most of the covariance with the outcome (Hadi and Ling 1998).

10.4.3 PLS Regression

PLS regression seeks to select components that maximise the covariance matrix between **y** and **t**. PLS extracts components that are also weighted combinations of the original p variables, but also takes into account their correlations with the outcome. In other words, in PCA, the extraction of components is independent of the outcome variables, whereas in PLS, components are extracted explicitly for their association with the outcome. The extraction of PLS components operates under the same constraints as with PCA: (1) the sum of the squared weights is unity; and (2) the correlations amongst all components are zero. When there are six covariates without perfect multicollinearity, six PLS components can be extracted (and they are independent of each other). PLS components are ordered according to the amount of variance in the outcome that is explained; that is, the first PLS component has a higher correlation with the outcome than the second PLS component, and the second has a higher correlation than the third, etc. In PLS, the first PLS component explains most of the outcome variance. For p variables, $x_1, x_2, ..., x_p$, each PLS component, $plsc_i$, is also a weighted composite of p covariates:

$$plsc_i = w_{i1}x_1 + w_{i2}x_2 + ... + w_{ip}x_p. \qquad (10.2)$$

The PLS regression coefficient for each x_i is derived from the sum of products of the regression coefficients for PLS components and the weight for each x_i. For example, when the outcome y is regressed on the first two PLS components, the equation is given as

$$y = \beta_1 * plsc_1 + \beta_2 * plsc_2 + \varepsilon$$

$$= \beta_1(w_{11}x_1 + w_{12}x_2 + ... + w_{1p}x_p) + \beta_2(w_{21}x_1 + w_{22}x_2 + ... + w_{2p}x_p) + \varepsilon$$

where β_1 and β_2 are the regression coefficients for PLS components 1 and 2, respectively, and ε is the residual error term. The PLS regression coefficient for x_1 is therefore $\beta_1 w_{11} + \beta_2 w_{21}$.

Note that if all six PLS components are used as new covariates, the results from the PLS regression, such as regression coefficients and R^2, are equivalent to those from PCA regression and OLS regression. The advantage of PLS over PCA is that the first few components explain most of the covariance between the outcome and covariates and, as a result, the caveat of PCA regression previously discussed does not occur in PLS regression.

10.4.4 PLS and Perfect Collinearity

As we explained in Chapter 6, when there is perfect collinearity in the data, one or more of the collinear variables have to be dropped for OLS to continue with its computations. From a statistical viewpoint, this is because the covariates data matrix does not have enough degrees of freedom; in statistical jargon, the matrix is not full rank. However, this is not a problem for either PCA or PLS regression.

Suppose we wish to estimate the effects of zwt_0, zwt_{19} and zwt_{19-0}, for instance. Since these three covariates are perfectly collinear, at least one of them has to be omitted for OLS regression as shown in Table 9.2 in Chapter 9. In PCA and PLS, perfect collinearity amongst the three variables means that only two components can be extracted from the three covariates, but each of the two components is *a combination of the original three variables*. From a statistical viewpoint, this is related to an important property in the singular value decomposition of a symmetric square matrix (see the next section for details). In OLS regression, the relation between the outcome SBP and zwt_0, zwt_{19} and zwt_{19-0} is given as

$$SBP = b_0 + b_1 zwt_0 + b_2 zwt_{19} + b_3 zwt_{19-0} + e, \qquad (10.3)$$

where b_0 is the intercept, b_1 is the regression coefficient for zwt_0, b_2 is the regression coefficient for zwt_{19}, b_3 regression coefficient for zwt_{19-0}, and e the residual error term. To obtain solutions for b_s requires the inversion of cross-product matrix for three covariates:

$$y = Xb + e \tag{10.4}$$

$$b = (X^TX)^{-1}X^Ty \tag{10.5}$$

In matrix algebra language, **b** is a vector for the three regression coefficients, **X** is an $n \times 3$ matrix (n is the number of subjects; e.g., $n = 834$ in our Cebu cohort), X^T is the transpose of **X**; that is, a $3 \times n$ matrix. The product matrix X^TX is therefore a 3×3 matrix, and if all three covariates are standardised variables with zero means and unit variances, this matrix divided by $(n - 1)$ is the correlation matrix for the three covariates. Therefore, Equation 10.4 can be expressed as

$$b = (n-1)R^{-1}X^Ty \tag{10.6}$$

$$R = \begin{bmatrix} 1 & r_1 & r_2 \\ r_1 & 1 & r_3 \\ r_2 & r_3 & 1 \end{bmatrix}$$

To estimate **b**, we need to obtain the inverse matrix of **R**, R^{-1}. The problem is that when **R** is not full rank (because, for example, variables in **R** are perfectly collinear), R^{-1} does not exist because the determinant of **R** is zero and the reciprocal of zero is infinity. This is why at least one of the perfectly collinear variables has to be dropped to ensure that the revised matrix **R** has a non-zero determinant. However, although R^{-1} does not exist, there is a generalised inverse matrix of **R**, and this is why PCA and PLS can work in data with perfectly collinear variables. Obtaining the generalised inverse matrix is related to the singular value decomposition of a square symmetric matrix, as explained in the next section.

10.4.5 Singular Value Decomposition, PCA and PLS Regression

To understand how singular value decomposition (SVD) works requires some knowledge of matrix algebra, and therefore, in this section, we will focus on the concept of SVD and its relation to regression analysis rather than its mathematical details. In the last section, we showed that to obtain OLS regression coefficients we need to invert the matrix X^TX or **R**. Both matrices are square; that is, its number of rows is equal to its number of columns. Also note that R (and also X^TX) is a symmetric matrix; that is, its first column is exactly the same as its first row, and its second column is exactly the same as its second row, etc. For any symmetric matrix (which must be square), it can be shown that it can be deconstructed into a product of three square matrices; that is,

$$R = U\Lambda U^T \tag{10.7}$$

The 3×3 matrix U contains the three eigenvectors of R, and U^T is the transpose of U (i.e., the rows in U become columns in U^T), and Λ is a 3×3 diagonal matrix such as

$$\Lambda = \begin{bmatrix} \lambda_1 & 0 & 0 \\ 0 & \lambda_2 & 0 \\ 0 & 0 & \lambda_3 \end{bmatrix},$$

where λ_1, λ_2 and λ_3 are eigenvalues of R. An important property of the three matrices is that the inverse of R is therefore the inverse of the product matrix $U\Lambda U^T$:

$$R^{-1} = (U\Lambda U^T)^{-1} = U^T\Lambda^{-1}U. \tag{10.8}$$

For the square matrix U with eigenvectors, its inverse matrix is just its transposed matrix. For the diagonal matrix Λ, its inverse is a matrix in which the diagonal elements are simply the reciprocal of the original elements; that is,

$$\Lambda^{-1} = \begin{bmatrix} 1/\lambda_1 & 0 & 0 \\ 0 & 1/\lambda_2 & 0 \\ 0 & 0 & 1/\lambda_3 \end{bmatrix}.$$

Suppose we only keep $1/\lambda_1$ in the matrix Λ^{-1} and replace $1/\lambda_2$ and $1/\lambda_3$ with zeros, the new matrix will become

$$\Lambda^{+1} = \begin{bmatrix} 1/\lambda_1 & 0 & 0 \\ 0 & 0 & 0 \\ 0 & 0 & 0 \end{bmatrix}$$

If we now substitute Λ^{-1} with Λ^{+1} in Equation 10.8 to obtain $R^{+1} = U^T\Lambda^{+1}U$, and then substitute R^{+1} in Equation 10.6 to obtain b^{+1},

$$b^{+1} = (n-1)R^{+1}X^Ty, \tag{10.9}$$

where the new set of regression coefficient $\mathbf{b}^{+1}$ is actually the PCA regression coefficients when the first PCA component is retained. If we keep $1/\lambda_1$ and $1/\lambda_2$ in the matrix Λ^{-1} and replace $1/\lambda_3$ with zero and thus create the new matrix Λ^{+2}, we will be able to obtain a new set of regression coefficient $\mathbf{b}^{+2}$, which is PCA regression coefficients with the first two PCA components retained. For PLS regression, the SVD analysis is carried out for $\mathbf{X}^{\mathsf{T}}\mathbf{y}$ in Equation 10.6, and as its procedure is more complex, we refer interested readers to consult a paper by Hoskuldsson (1988).

For matrices without full rank, it is still possible to undertake SVD analysis. For instance, when $\mathbf{R}$ is the correlation matrix for zwt_0, zwt_{19} and zwt_{19-0}, there are only two eigenvalues in Λ:

$$\Lambda = \begin{bmatrix} \lambda_1 & 0 & 0 \\ 0 & \lambda_2 & 0 \\ 0 & 0 & 0 \end{bmatrix}$$

The generalised inverse of Λ is given as

$$\Lambda^+ = \begin{bmatrix} 1/\lambda_1 & 0 & 0 \\ 0 & 1/\lambda_2 & 0 \\ 0 & 0 & 0 \end{bmatrix}$$

Therefore, whilst it is not possible to regress SBP on zwt_0, zwl_{19} and zwt_{19-0} using OLS regression, it is possible to use PCA or PLS regression. A more detailed and also more technical explanation about SVD and generalised inverse in regression analysis can be found in Mandel (1982). A non-technical explanation about how PCA and PLS work for perfectly collinear variables can be found in our recent publication (Tu et al. 2010).

Phatak and De Jong (1997) provided an interesting and enlightening geometric explanation for PLS regression. In Figure 10.2, $\mathbf{y}_p$ is the projection of the outcome $\mathbf{y}$ onto the plane spanned by the covariate vectors $\mathbf{x}_1$ and $\mathbf{x}_2$. The ellipse S is the PCA space spanned by the two principal components, $\mathbf{pc}_1$ and $\mathbf{pc}_2$. S is an ellipse because the sum of squared weights in Equation 10.1 is constrained to unity; that is, S encompasses all vectors $\mathbf{t}$ that have the unity length (as $\mathbf{x}_1$ and $\mathbf{x}_2$ are standardised vectors) and satisfy $\mathbf{t} = w_1\mathbf{x}_1 + w_2\mathbf{x}_2$ and $w_1^2 + w_2^2 = 1$.

Since PLS components are under the same constraint for their weights, PLS components are also within S. The task is to find the vector $\mathbf{t}$ in S that has the largest covariance with $\mathbf{y}$. As $\mathbf{y}_p$ is the orthogonal project of $\mathbf{y}$, this is equivalent to finding a vector $\mathbf{t}$ in S with the largest covariance with $\mathbf{y}_p$. In terms of vector geometry, to find the vector $\mathbf{t}$, we draw a line l, which is perpendicular to $\mathbf{y}_p$ and move it toward S until it connects S with T; that is, l is now a tangent to S. The vector $\overline{OT}$ (O is the origin) is then the first PLS

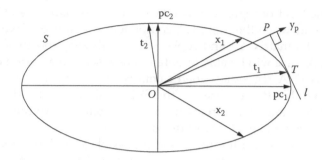

FIGURE 10.2
Geometrical presentation of PLS regression.

component t_1, as any other vectors in S has a smaller covariance with y_p. The covariance between t_1 and y_p is $\overline{OP}$, where P is the intersection between l and y_p. The second PLS component t_2 is the vector in S that is orthogonal to t_1. A few observations can be made about Figure 10.2:

1. When y_p is projected on pca1, $t_1 = \mathbf{pc}_1$. Consequently, PCA and PLS will have the same results. When y_p is projected on pca2, $t_1 = \mathbf{pc}_2$, and $\mathbf{pc}_1$ explains no variance in y.

2. The total variance in y that can be explained by x_1 and x_2 is always the same for OLS, PCA and PLS regression because the space into which y is projected is the same.

3. PLS components may be viewed as a rotation of principal components where the first component has the largest covariance with y_p amongst all vectors in the space S.

10.4.6 Selection of PLS Component

As explained in the previous section, PCA seeks to maximise the variance of each component, and the selection of the PCA component is based on either the values of components (such as the criterion eigenvalues > 1) or the diminishing decline in variances amongst the covariates (as indicated by the scree plot). PLS seeks to maximise the covariance between the outcome and new composites, so it seems justifiable to use the increments in the explained variance in the outcome (e.g., changes in R^2) as a criterion for selecting PLS components. This gives us a measure of predictive ability, the predictive residual error sum of squares (PRESS; Wakeling and Morris 1993). To obtain this, the data are first split into a number of groups, and for each a prediction is obtained using the model derived from all other groups. For example, one observation is left out of the model, and we use the remaining observations to predict the outcome. PRESS is calculated as the sum of squares of the differences between the prediction for each observation (when it is left out of the model) and the observed value of the dependent variables. A problem we address is that, while a small value of PRESS indicates internal consistency of the model, it is not a guarantee that a real effect has been observed (Wakeling and Morris 1993; Wold et al. 2001; Abdi 2010).

Another index is Q^2, the cross-validated R^2. In OLS regression, R^2 is calculated as

$$R^2 = \left(1 - \left(\frac{\text{RSS}}{\text{SS}}\right)\right),$$

where RSS is the residual sum of squares and SS is the sum of squares; that is, (RSS/SS) is the proportion of the outcome not explained by the model, and therefore R^2 is the proportion of the outcome explained by the model. The formula for Q^2 is very similar to R^2:

$$Q^2 = \left(1 - \left(\frac{\text{PRESS}}{\text{SS}}\right)\right).$$

For selecting the PLS component, we can calculate the improvement in Q^2 as a ratio:

$$Q_p^2 \text{Imp} = \frac{Q_p^2 - Q_{p-1}^2}{Q_{p-1}^2}.$$

Usually, an arbitrary value, for example, 0.05, is set, which corresponds to a 5% improvement (Abdi 2010).

10.4.7 PLS Regression for Lifecourse Data Using Weight z-Scores at Birth, Changes in z-Scores, and Current Weight z-Scores

For PLS regression analysis, *SBP* is first regressed on zwt_0, zwt_{19} and zwt_{19-0}, and then regressed simultaneously on zwt_0, the five successive weight z-scores increments, and zwt_{19}. We used a free data-mining software package *Tanagra* (http://eric.univ-lyon2.fr/~ricco/tanagra/en/tanagra.html) for PLS regression analyses because it has a well-organised output. PLS regression can also be undertaken using standard statistical software packages such as SAS® (SAS Institute, Inc., Cary, NC) or the library pls in *R* (R Foundation for Statistical Computing, Vienna, Austria). Note that, due to different default settings for variables scaling, PLS analysis output may look slightly different using different packages. For example, although SAS and Tanagra give the same PLS regression coefficients, SAS reports different weights; that is, w_{ij} in Equation 10.2. The weights reported by Tanagra (Lyon 2003) are eigenvectors with the length of each vector equal to unity. In contrast, SAS does not scale the weight vectors to have unit length. As no distributional assumption is made for PLS regression coefficients, their confidence intervals are usually obtained using resampling methods such as the bootstrap or jacknife method.

The bootstrap method in PLS seeks to generate new data sets from the collected sample. For example, suppose we have 200 observations in the sample. When we randomly select the first observation, say number 50, from our sample, we put it back and then randomly select the second observation until we obtain 200 observations for the new data set. Note that as each observation when selected is replaced, some may be selected more than once (otherwise, the new data set will be exactly the same as the original). We repeat this process many times and then run the same PLS analysis for each new data set. Therefore, we shall have a distribution of each parameter, such as weights and loadings, for our model. Jacknife does resampling differently by leaving one observation out of the sample each time and running the PLS analysis on the remaining sample (Chin 1999). In this chapter we calculate 95% CIs using 500 bootstrap replications.

When SBP is regressed on the first PLS component extracted from the covariates zwt_0, zwt_{19-0} and zwt_{19}, associations between the outcome and each covariate were similar to those in the bivariate OLS regression. Table 10.3 shows that both zwt_{19} and zwt_{19-0} had positive associations with SBP, whilst zwt_0 showed no such association. When two components were extracted and used as covariates in PLS regression, there were only small changes in the regression coefficients. More than 97% of the covariance between the outcome and the three variables were explained by the first PLS component. Therefore, the analysis based on a single component is sufficient and appropriate.

When SBP is regressed on the first PLS component of zwt_0, the five successive weight z-score increments and zwt_{19}, zwt_{19} yield a positive association with SBP, whilst zwt_0 has a small negative association (Table 10.3). Early changes in weight z-scores have relatively small positive associations with the outcome compared to later growth in weight z-scores. Adding further PLS components to the model hardly affects the coefficients, and the zwt_0 coefficient becomes statistically significant. Growth from birth to age 2 years has a relatively smaller positive effect on SBP compared to later growth from age 8 to 19 years. Most of the covariance between SBP and the seven variables is explained by the first PLS component, and the coefficients for the seven covariates in the model with two components only showed very small changes as additional components were added. This suggests that there are only two dimensions to the data. Figures 10.3 is a graphical presentation of the PLS regression coefficients of models for different numbers of components for SBP. The effect of growth increases with age, but current body size has the greatest effect in predicting blood pressure.

10.4.8 The Relationship between OLS Regression and PLS Regression Coefficients

PLS estimates the individual contribution of birth, growth and current body size to the prediction of blood pressure, and there is a mathematical

TABLE 10.3

Results from Partial Least Squares Regression with Three Body Size Measurements or with Seven Body Size Measurements as Covariates for 834 Girls. The Outcome Variable Is Systolic Blood Pressure (*SBP*) at Age 19 Years.

Components	1		2		3	
	Coefficient	95% CI	Coefficient	95% CI	Coefficient	95% CI
zwt_0	−0.29	(−0.66, 0.09)	−0.14	(−0.59, 0.32)		
zwt_{19-0}	0.91	(0.60, 1.21)	0.88	(0.57, 1.17)		
zwt_{19}	1.05	(0.64, 1.45)	1.15	(0.69, 1.57)		
$CumR^2$	4.76%		4.81%			
zwt_0	−0.38	(−0.92, 0.10)	−0.60	(−1.11, −0.09)	−0.61	(−1.18, −0.09)
zwt_{1-0}	0.26	(−0.15, 0.69)	0.24	(−0.15, 0.64)	0.19	(−0.22, 0.65)
zwt_{2-1}	0.11	(−0.78, 1.01)	0.56	(−0.56, 1.58)	0.59	(−0.53, 1.59)
zwt_{8-2}	0.33	(−0.22, 0.81)	0.13	(−0.52, 0.74)	0.18	(−0.50, 0.78)
zwt_{15-8}	1.31	(0.55, 2.10)	1.58	(0.70, 2.42)	1.59	(0.73, 2.41)
zwt_{19-15}	1.43	(0.56, 2.17)	1.48	(0.54, 2.43)	1.53	(0.58, 2.48)
zwt_{19}	1.37	(0.89, 1.82)	1.30	(0.77, 1.80)	1.28	(0.74, 1.81)
$CumR^2$	5.78%		6.01%		6.02%	

Components	4		5		6	
	Coefficient	95% CI	Coefficient	95% CI	Coefficient	95% CI
zwt_0						
zwt_{19-0}						
zwt_{19}						
$CumR^2$						
zwt_0	−0.63	(−1.17, −0.10)	−0.62	(−1.17, −0.10)	−0.62	(−1.17, −0.10)
zwt_{1-0}	0.19	(−0.24, 0.64)	0.19	(−0.23, 0.64)	0.19	(−0.23, 0.64)
zwt_{2-1}	0.57	(−0.55, 1.59)	0.57	(−0.56, 1.59)	0.57	(−0.56, 1.59)
zwt_{8-2}	0.18	(−0.49, 0.79)	0.18	(−0.49, 0.79)	0.18	(−0.49, 0.79)
zwt_{15-8}	1.59	(0.73, 2.42)	1.59	(0.73, 2.42)	1.59	(0.73, 2.42)
zwt_{19-15}	1.53	(0.57, 2.48)	1.54	(0.57, 2.48)	1.54	(0.57, 2.48)
zwt_{19}	1.27	(0.74, 1.80)	1.27	(0.74, 1.80)	1.27	(0.74, 1.80)
$CumR^2$	6.02%		6.02%		6.02%	

Note: The number of components means how many PLS components were extracted as covariates in the regression analysis. $CumR^2$ is the cumulative R^2 explained by the number of components.

relationship between PLS results with full dimension (the maximum number of components retained) and OLS regression coefficients. For instance, when *SBP* is regressed on zwt_0, zwt_{19-0} and zwt_{19}, the equation for the PLS model with two components is given as (Table 10.3)

$$SBP = -0.14zwt_0 + 0.88zwt_{19-0} + 1.15zwt_{19}.$$

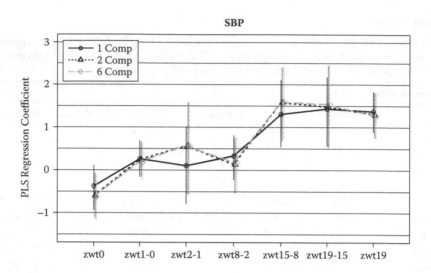

FIGURE 10.3
Graphical presentation of PLS regression coefficients for *SBP* regressed on one, two or six PLS components. The covariates are the seven variables for birth weight z-score, five successive z-score weight increments and current body weight z-score.

Simple rearrangements can give rise to OLS regression models with two of the three covariates (the differences in the second decimal is due to rounding errors):

$$SBP = -0.14zwt_0 + 0.88(zwt_{19} - zwt_0) + 1.15zwt_{19}$$

$$SBP = (-0.14 - 0.88)zwt_0 + (0.88 + 1.15)zwt_{19}$$

$$SBP = -1.02zwt_0 + 2.03zwt_{19}.$$

[OLS multivariable regression 2 in Table 10.1]

The other two multivariable regression models in Table 10.1 can be derived in a similar way.

For *SBP* regressed on zwt_0, the five successive weight z-score increments and zwt_{19}, simple rearrangements by replacing zwt_{19} with ($zwt_0 + zwt_{1-0} + zwt_{2-1} + zwt_{8-2} + zwt_{15-8} + zwt_{19-15}$) can give rise to OLS multivariable regression 1, and by replacing zwt_0 with ($zwt19 - zwt_{1-0} - zwt_{2-1} - zwt_{8-2} - zwt_{15-8} - zwt_{19-15}$) can lead to OLS multivariable regression 2 in Table 10.2.

From a geometrical point of view, this is because the least squares projection of the outcome vector **y** onto the space spanned by the covariates is the same vector **ŷ** as that in PCA or PLS regression when the maximum number of components are retained (as we explained in the previous section, these three methods will have the same R^2). Therefore, OLS regression coefficients can always be derived from PCA or PLS as long as the outcome is projected onto the same covariate space. For example, the covariate space spanned by zwt_0 and zwt_{19} is the same as that spanned by zwt_0, zwt_{19-0} and zwt_{19}.

10.4.9 PLS Regression for Lifecourse Data Using Weight z-Scores Measured at Six Different Ages

In Section 10.4.7, *SBP* is regressed on z-score birth weight, z-score current weight and five successive z-score increments in PLS analysis. An alternative approach would be to undertake PLS analysis on the original six z-score weights, which can be viewed as the PLS version of lifecourse plots (e.g., Figure 9.6 in Chapter 9). As the six variables are highly correlated (up to 0.82 in Table 9.1), collinearity is a potential problem for OLS regression, confirmed in our analysis in which there are negative associations between blood pressure and birth weight, weight at 1 year or 2 years, and large regression coefficients for weight at 18 years (Figure 10.4). It is also noted that the CI for regression coefficients in the PLS model with one component are much smaller than those in the PLS model with six components. PLS analysis shows that the model with only two components was required to achieve most of the model R^2, and the indices for component selection (such as improvement in Q^2 and PRESS) suggest that the model with the first component is the most parsimonious. The association between body weights and blood pressure increases with age, whilst early body weights have non-significant negative associations in models with two or more components (Figure 10.4).

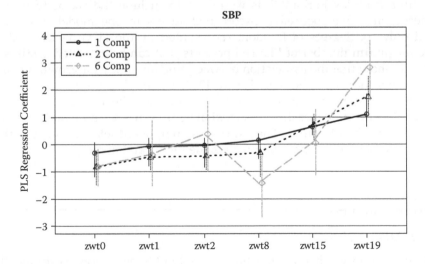

FIGURE 10.4
Graphical presentation of PLS regression coefficients for *SBP* regressed on one, two or six PLS components. The covariates are the six original body weight z-scores.

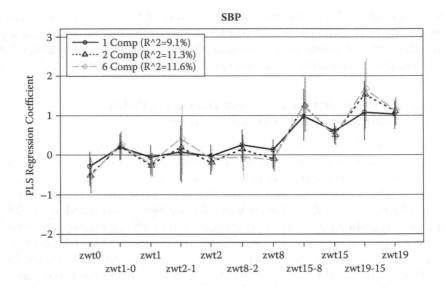

FIGURE 10.5
Graphical presentation of PLS regression coefficients for *SBP* regressed on one, two or six PLS components. The covariates are the six original body weight z-scores and the five successive z-score weight increments.

10.4.10 PLS Regression for Lifecourse Data Using Weight *z*-Scores Measured at Six Different Ages and Five Changes in *z*-Scores

A more complex PLS analysis would be to include the six body weight z-scores and five successive z-score increments in one model. There are still only six degrees of freedom represented by the 11 variables; that is, the maximum number of PLS components that can be extracted is still six. Results show that the association between *SBP* and body (or growth in) size in general increases with age (Figure 10.5). Although the zigzag courses in the plots seem to indicate that collinearity may still be a concern, there is a general trend in the positive associations between age and blood pressure throughout the lifecourse. The indices for component selection suggest that the model with only one component is the most parsimonious.

10.5 Discussion

In this chapter we demonstrate how to apply PLS regression to estimate the effects of body weights and growth in weights at different stages throughout the lifecourse. PLS analysis reveals that birth weight has a negligible effect on *SBP*, and current body weight has the largest effect. Growth in later childhood and adolescence has a stronger association with *SBP* than earlier growth.

When only one PLS component is extracted, associations between later-life blood pressure and the original covariates remain in the same direction, though with smaller values, as with standard OLS regression. Whilst OLS regression coefficients are unbiased estimates of the effect size, their confidence intervals increase with the degree of collinearity amongst covariates. In contrast, PLS regression provides *biased* (i.e., shrunken) estimates with smaller confidence intervals. The use of shrinkage regression methods (e.g., PLS, PCA and ridge regression) provide a trade-off between bias and precision (S. Wold et al. 2001; Hastie et al. 2009). In our illustration, the first PLS component explained most of the covariance between *SBP* and lifecourse body size measurements. Figure 10.2, which may be interpreted as an alternative presentation of the lifecourse plot (Cole 2004, 2007), shows that the curves from models with one PLS component are a good approximation to those from models with two or six components, and differences between the curves from the two- or six-component models are very small. The PLS model with two components may therefore be considered as the most parsimonious representation of each child's growth curve in relation to later-life *SBP*.

When there is perfect collinearity amongst covariates, there are, as shown in our illustration, simple relationships between PLS and OLS regression coefficients when the maximal number of components are extracted in PLS. Whilst the OLS regression coefficients can be obtained from PLS analysis, it is *not* possible to obtain PLS results from the OLS analysis because OLS analysis is unable to estimate the individual contribution of perfectly collinear variables. Moreover, the traditional OLS regression analysis of the adjustment of multiple body sizes will inevitably allocate the effects of lifecourse growth on later health inadequately. For example, the much larger positive effects for birth and growth in multivariable regression 1 in Tables 10.1 and 10.2 is caused by attributing the effects of current body size to the preceding body size measurements.

PLS may be viewed as an approach to distribute the overall contribution of body size and growth measurements to the outcomes according to the correlations amongst the covariates and between all covariates and the outcome. For example, current body size had the strongest association with *SBP* in our data set, and it is therefore not surprising that it also had large regression coefficients in PLS analysis, which are, however, smaller than the OLS estimates. PLS regression coefficients for later growth, such as zwt_{19-15}, were also smaller than the OLS estimates, indicating that some of the effects in OLS regression might be explained by girls with greater growth during these ages being more likely to become bigger adults. As body growth is a continuous process, measurements of body size at different ages, or growth in different phases during the lifecourse, are inevitably correlated, and these correlations are greater when the time interval between measurements is short. Therefore, it is intrinsically difficult to disentangle the lifecourse effects of growth on later-life health when analysing highly collinear lifecourse data using OLS and similarly limited standard regression methods, and this is why alternative methods, such as PLS regression, are required.

PLS is a dimension reduction method and, therefore, in general, not all PLS components are selected as covariates for regression analysis, as the first few PLS components usually explain most of the covariance between the outcome and covariates in the OLS regression. Otherwise, results from PLS regression would be the same as OLS regression, unless some of the original covariates are perfectly collinear. However, the more components selected as covariates, the greater the explained variance in y (i.e., the greater the model R^2); it is therefore essential to determine the appropriate complexity of the model; that is, we need to consider the balance between gain in model prediction and potential overfitting (S. Wold et al. 2001). For our example data set, from a statistical viewpoint, it seems sufficient to select the first component only since the remaining five explain <1% of total model R^2 for *SBP*, and this is confirmed by statistical indices such as PRESS and improvement in Q^2. However, as the major advantage of using PLS in lifecourse epidemiology over OLS regression is to estimate the effects of growth in different phases on health in later life, by overcoming the problem of perfect collinearity, the selection of the number of components should not be solely based on increases in the model R^2 or other similar indices.

10.6 Conclusion

In Chapters 9 and 10 we compare results from several statistical approaches to estimating the effects of growth during the lifecourse on health outcomes in later life. Although these approaches were intended to answer the same broad research question/hypothesis, there are nevertheless some subtle differences in what each approach does. Therefore, to choose *the best* analytical strategy requires further elaboration and clarification of the research question. For example, if the aim is to identify the growth pattern related to the higher risk of diseases in later life, group-based modelling and growth mixture modelling discussed in Chapter 9 are the preferred approaches. If the aim is to estimate the effects of growth at different phases throughout the lifecourse, latent growth curve models and partial least squares regression seem to be a better choice of analytical strategy.

Moreover, given the potential complexity in growth processes throughout the lifecourse, each statistical method (no matter how sophisticated) can only unravel some of the intricacies. For example, group-based modelling and growth mixture modelling are useful because characteristics of growth patterns are estimated and their associations with disease outcomes are explored. Whilst these methods are powerful tools in identifying distinct growth patterns, it is well known that these methods do not always provide stable results due to problems in model convergence around local maxima/ minima (Bauer 2007) and sometimes it is not straightforward to determine the optimal or *true* number of classes or trajectories in the sample data. It would also be more difficult to compare growth patterns uncovered in different data sets using these methods than to compare PLS regression coefficients, and therefore more difficult to validate or corroborate results across different studies and populations. Furthermore, unlike any likelihood-based methods, such as structural equation modelling, PLS algorithms always achieve convergence and are free from problems of inadmissible results, such as the Heywood cases (Dillon et al. 1987). This makes PLS a useful tool in exploring lifecourse effects of growth in body size on later-life health outcomes. Recent developments in PLS have been extended to generalised linear models (Chevalier et al. 2006). PLS can also be used in research where collinearity may be a major problem, such as analysing the associations between components in metabolic syndrome and health outcomes in later life. PLS path modelling, an alternative approach to structural equation modelling, can also be useful to medical and epidemiological research due to its ability to deal with collinearity and small samples. An example of PLS path modelling in dental research can be found in our recent paper (Tu et al. 2009b).

11

Concluding Remarks

In this book we have sought to provide some insight into how one might conceptualise the statistical problems encountered in epidemiology using practical examples that prevail in contemporary epidemiological research. Some of the focus has been related to lifecourse epidemiology, as this is the main area of research that interests both authors. However, from a more heuristic statistical viewpoint, it could be said that the main focus has been somewhat that of the evaluation of the effects caused by environmental exposure and interventions within a non-randomised, that is, observational, setting. It is the often challenging setting of observational research where context becomes key, since, in the absence of experiments, confounding and many other potentially distorting influences can operate to affect the statistical interpretation central to addressing research questions. It is the emphasis on this problem, that is, the interpretation of empirical research evidence, the need to respect and therefore reflect upon context, per se and the need to consider carefully all implications and limitations of the statistical methods used in observational research that we have dedicated this book to.

As emphasised at the outset, this does not mean that our thinking is always correct, that our interpretation is always right, or that our approach is definitive and the best. What we have sought, however, is to present an honest disclosure of our detailed thoughts and an indication of our views that have emerged from our research deliberations. We feel that there is a huge gap in the literature for postgraduate students and junior researchers to develop their research skills: on the one hand, journal articles are usually written in the standard *introduction-materials* and *methods-results-discussion* format, with the least space given to the introduction, where the authors describe why they investigate the particular issues and how they develop their thinking in solving those issues; on the other hand, most textbooks focus on explaining the mathematics behind specific statistical methods and using some very simple examples to test overtly straightforward research hypothesis. However, in observational research, any research hypothesis is just a node in a network of hypotheses within a broader biological theory. To test one hypothesis in isolation usually requires making strong assumptions about other hypotheses in the same network. This book is to bridge the gap by paying greater attention to the development of thinking before embarking upon the statistical analyses.

In this book we have touched upon sometimes diverse and sometimes related statistical issues, but the principles of thinking outside the box, or merely questioning received wisdom, is an overriding principle that applies to all applications of statistics, and not just observational biomedical research. We therefore cannot hope to cover all problems and pitfalls in the use of statistics in biomedical research; indeed, it is likely that many remain as yet unrealised, or undiscovered, in the sense that someone is yet to point out the limitations of certain methods in certain contexts. Many such limitations may seem obvious (to some) after the event, though some may remain controversial, as with some of the issues we have tackled in this book. Such problems often need methodological developments to advance the application of statistics, whilst some issues remain unresolved and may only be settled when the biological and physiological mechanisms are well understood.

It is also worth noting that the type of issues we outline in this book is not unique to biomedical research. The journey toward discovering some of the pitfalls in applied statistics, as outlined in this book, has been a varied path and has covered many a diverse subject domains. It is thus important to recognise that what we have sought to address in principle, that is, to promote the need for careful statistical thinking in the application of statistical methods in biomedical research, is just as relevant to other applied domains. For instance, in social sciences, such as economics, education and psychology, observational research is the norm, as it is usually infeasible or unethical to undertake randomised controlled trials. Discussions of many issues we address in this book can be found in the literature in those areas. Our hope, therefore, is that the philosophical message of this book is transferable to other fields and it is just as relevant that the applied statistician in any of the aforementioned disciplines can read this book. In any event, we hope we have cast some light on some of the mysteries and confusions that prevail in the application of statistics to observational research, particularly within biomedicine.

References

Abdi, H. (2010). Partial least squares regression and projection on latent structure regression (PLS regression). *WIREs Computational Statistics*. **2**, 97–106.

Adair, L. (2007). Size at birth and growth trajectories to young adulthood. *American Journal of Human Biology*. **19**, 327–337.

Adair, L.S., Cole, T.J. (2005). Rapid child growth raises blood pressure in adolescent boys who were thin at birth. *Hypertension*. **41**, 451–456.

Aldrich, J. (1995). Correlation genuine and spurious in Pearson and Yule. *Statistical Science*. **10**, 364–376.

Altman, D.G. (1982). Statistics in medical journals. *Statistics in Medicine*. **1**, 59–71.

Altman, D.G. (1991a). *Practical Statistics for Medical Research*. London: Chapman and Hall/CRC.

Altman, D.G. (1991b). Statistics in medical journals: Developments in the 1980s. *Statistics in Medicine*. **10**, 1897–1913.

Altman, D.G. (1994). Letter to the editor: Problems in dichotomizing continuous variables. *American Journal of Epidemiology*. **139**, 442.

Altman, D.G., Lausen, B., Sauerbrei, W., Schmacher, M. (1994). Dangers of using "optimal" cutpoints in the evaluation of prognostic factors. *Journal of the National Cancer Institute*. **86**, 829–835.

Andersen, B. (1990). *Methodological Errors in Medical Research*. London: Blackwell.

Arah, O. (2008). The role of causal reasoning in understanding Simpson's paradox, Lord's paradox, and the suppression effect: Covariate selection in the analysis of observational studies. *Emerging Themes in Epidemiology*. **5**, 5.

Archie, J.P. (1981). Mathematical Coupling: A common source of error. *Annals of Surgery*. **193**, 296–303.

Baker, G.A. (1942). Correlations between functions of variables. *Journal of American Statistical Association*. **37**, 537–539.

Barker, D.J. (2004). Developmental origins of adult health and disease. *Journal of Epidemiology and Community Health*. **58**, 114–115.

Barker, D.J.P. (1996). The fetal origins of hypertension. *Journal of Hypertension*. **14**, S117–S120.

Barker, D.J.P. (2001). *Fetal Origins of Cardiovascular and Lung Disease*. New York: Marcel Dekker.

Barker, D.J.P. (2003). The midwife, the coincidence, and the hypothesis. *British Medical Journal*. **327**, 1428–1430.

Barker, D.J.P., Bull, A.R., Osmond, C., et al. (1990). Fetal and placental size and risk of hypertension in adult life. *British Medical Journal*. **301**, 259–62.

Barker, D.J.P., Osmond, C. (1986). Infant mortality, childhood nutrition, and ischaemic heart disease in England and Wales. *The Lancet*. **i**, 1077–1081.

Barker, D.J.P., Osmond, C., Forsen, T.J. Kajantie, E., Eriksson, J.G. (2005). Trajectories of growth among children who have coronary events as adults. *New England Journal of Medicine*. **353**, 1802–1809.

Barker, D.J.P., Winter, P.D., Osmond, C., et al. (1989). Weight in infancy and death from ischaemic heart disease. *The Lancet*. **ii**, 577–80.

Barros, F.C., Victora, C.G. (1999). Increased blood pressure in adolescents who were small for gestational age at birth: A cohort study in Brazil. *International Journal Epidemiology.* **28**, 676–681.

Bartko, J.J., Pettigrew, K. (1968). A note on the correlation of parts with wholes. *The American Statistician.* **22**, 41.

Bauer, D.J. (2007). Observations on the use of growth mixture models in psychological research. *Multivariate Behavioral Research.* **42**, 757–786.

Belsley, D.A. (1991). *Conditioning Diagnostics: Collinearity and Weak Data in Regression.* New York: Wiley.

Ben-Shlomo, Y., Kuh, D. (2002). A life course approach to chronic disease epidemiology: Conceptual models, empirical challenges and interdisciplinary perspectives. *International Journal of Epidemiology.* **31**, 285–93.

Bhargava, S.K., Sachdev, H.S., Fall, C.H.D., Osmond, C., Lakshmy, R., Barker, D.J.P., Biswas, S.K.D., Ramji, S., Prabhakaran, D., Reddy, K.S. (2004). Relation of serial changes in childhood body-mass index to impaired glucose tolerance in young adulthood. *New England Journal of Medicine.* **350**, 865–875.

Blance, A., Tu, Y.-K., Gilthorpe, M.S. (2005). A multilevel modelling solution to mathematical coupling. *Statistical Methods in Medical Research.* **14**, 553–565.

Bland, J.M., Altman, D.G. (1994a). Regression towards the mean. *British Medical Journal.* **308**, 1499.

Bland, J.M., Altman, D.G. (1994b). Some examples of regression towards the mean. *British Medical Journal.* **309**, 780.

Blomqvist, N. (1977). On the relation between change and initial value. *Journal of the American Statistical Association.* **72**, 746–749.

Blomqvist, N. (1987). On the bias caused by regression towards the mean. *Journal of Clinical Periodontology.* **13**, 34–37.

Blomqvist, N., Dahlen, G. (1985). Analysis of change-are baseline measurements needed? *Journal of Clinical Periodontology.* **12**, 877–881.

Bollen, K.A. (1989). *Structural Equations with Latent Variables.* New York: Wiley.

Bollen, K.A., Curran, P.J. (2006). *Latent Curve Models.* Hoboken, NJ: Wiley.

Bonate, P. (2000). *Analysis of Pretest–Posttest Designs.* Boca Raton, FL: Chapman & Hall/CRC.

Boshuizen, H.C. (2005). Letter to the editor. *Journal of Clinical Epidemiology.* **58**, 209–210.

Boulesteix, A.L., Strimmer, K. (2007). Partial least squares: A versatile tool for the analysis of high-dimensional genomic data. *Brief in Bioinformatics.* **8**, 32–44.

Brand, R. (1994). Author's reply: Importance of trends in the interpretation of an overall odds ratio in the meta-analysis of clinical trials. *Statistics in Medicine.* **13**, 295–296.

Bray, J.H., Maxwell, S.E. (1985). *Multivariate Analysis of Variance.* Sage University Paper Series on Quantitative Applications in the Social Sciences, 07-054. Newbury Park, CA: Sage.

Bring, J. (1996). A geometric approach to compare variables in a regression model. *The American Statistician.* **50**, 57–62.

Burke, V., Beilin, L.J., Blake, K.V., Doherty, D., Kendall, G.E., Newnham, L.I., Stanley, F.J. (2004). Indicators of foetal growth do not independently predict blood pressure in 8-year-old Australians: A prospective cohort study. *Hypertension.* **43**, 208–213.

Campbell, D.T., Kenny, D.A. (1999). *A Primer on Regression Artifacts.* New York: The Guilford Press.

Carlsson, S., Persson, P.-G., Alvarsson, M., Efendic, S., Norman, A., Svanstrom, L., Ostenson, C.G., Grill, V. (1999). Low birth weight, family history of diabetes, and glucose intolerance in Swedish middle-aged men. *Diabetes Care.* **22**, 1043–1047.

Carroll, J.D., Green, P.E., Chaturvedi, A. (1997). *Mathematical Tools for Applied Multivariate Analysis*, revised edition. San Diego: Academic Press.

Ceesay, S.M., Prentice, A.M., Cole, T.J., Foord, F., Poskitt, E.M.E., Weaver, L.T., Whitehead, R.G. (1997). Effects on birth weight and perinatal mortality of maternal dietary supplements in rural Gambia: 5 Year randomised controlled trial. *British Medical Journal.* **315**, 786–790.

Chatterjee, S., Hadi, A.S., Price, B. (2006). *Regression Analysis by Example*, 4th ed. New York: John Wiley & Sons.

Chevallier, S., Bertrand, D., Kohler, A., Courcoux, P. (2006). Application of PLS-DA in multivariate image analysis. *Journal of Chemometrics.* **20**, 221–229.

Chin, W.W. (1999). The partial least squares approach for structural equation modeling. In Marcoulides, G.A., *Modern Methods for Business Research*. Mahwah, NJ: Lawrence Erlbaum Associates. pp. 295–336.

Cleary, P.J. (1986). L.I.V. R.I.P.?: Comments on Myrtek and Foerster's 'The Law of Initial Value: A Rare Exception'. *Biological Psychology.* **22**, 279–284.

Cohen, J., Cohen, P. (1983). *Applied Multiple Regression/Correlation Analysis for the Behavioral Sciences*. 2nd ed. Hillsdale: LEA.

Cole, T. (2007). The life course plot in life course analysis. In Pickles, A., Maughan, B., Wadsworth, M., editors. *Epidemiological Methods in Life Course Research*. Oxford: Oxford University Press, pp. 137–155.

Cole, T.J. (2004). Modeling postnatal exposures and their interactions with birth size. *Journal of Nutrition.* **134**, 201–204.

Cole, T.J. (2005). Letter to the editor. *American Journal of Epidemiology.* **162**, 394–395.

Cortellini, P., Tonetti, M.S. (2000). Focus on intrabony defects: Guided tissue regeneration. *Periodontology 2000.* **22**, 104–132.

Cox, D.R. (1957). Note on grouping. *Journal of the American Statistical Association.* **52**, 543–547.

Cox, D.R., Small, N.J.H. (1978). Testing multivariate normality. *Biometrika.* **65**, 263–272.

Cox, D.R., Wermuth, N. (1994). Tests of linearity, multivariate normality and the adequacy of linear scores. *Applied Statistics.* **43**, 347–355.

Cuadras, C.M. (1998). Letter to the editor. *The American Statistician.* **52**, 371.

Cumsille, F., Bangdiwala, S.I., Sen, P.K., Kupper, L.L. (2000). Effect of dichotomising a continuous variable on the model structure in multiple linear regression models. *Communications in Statistics—Theory and Method.* **29**, 643–654.

Curhan, G.C., Chertow, G.M., Willett, W.C., Spiegelman, D., Colditz, G.A., Manson, J.E., Speizer, F.E., Stampfer, M.J. (1996a). Birth weight and adult hypertension and obesity in women. *Circulation.* **94**, 1310–1315.

Curhan, G.C., Willett, W.C., Rimm, E.B., Spiegelman, D., Ascherio, A.L., Stampfer, M.J. (1996b). Birth weight and adult hypertension, diabetes mellitus, and obesity in US men. *Circulation.* **94**, 3246–3250.

Dahley, D.L., Adair, L.S., Bollen, K.A. (2009). A structural equation model of the developmental origins of blood pressure. *International Journal of Epidemiology.* **38**, 538–548.

Davies, A.A., Davey Smith, G., Ben-Shlomo, Y., Litchfield, P. (2004). Low birth weight is associated with higher adult total cholesterol concentration in men: Findings from an occupational cohort of 25843 employees. *Circulation.* **110**, 1258–1262.

Dawson, B., Trapp, R.G. (2001). *Basic and Clinical Biostatistics*, 3rd ed. New York: McGraw-Hill.

De Stavola, B.L., Nitsch, D., dos Santos Silva, I., et al. (2006). Statistical issues in life course epidemiology. *American Journal of Epidemiology*. **163**, 84–96.

de Jong, S. (1993). SIMPLS: An alternative approach to partial least squares regression. *Chemometrics and Intelligent Laboratory Systems*. **18**, 251–263.

Dillon, W.R., Kumar, A., Mulani, N. (1987). Offending estimates in covariance structure analysis: Comments on the causes of and solutions to Heywood cases. *Psychological Bulletin*. **101**, 126–135.

Draper, N.R., Smith, H. (1998). *Applied Regression Analysis*, 3rd ed. New York: John Wiley & Sons.

Duncan, T.E., Duncan, S.C., Strycker, L.A. (2006). *An Introduction to Latent Variable Growth Curve Modeling*, 2nd ed. Mahwah, NJ: Lawrence Erlbaum Associates.

Dunn, G. (2004). *Statistical Evaluation of Measurement Errors*, 2nd ed. London: Arnold.

Egger, M., Davey Smith, G., Altman, D.G. (2001). *Systematic Review in Health Care: Meta-Analysis in Context*. London: BMJ Publishing Group.

Ekstrom, D., Quade, D., Golden, R.N. (1990). Statistical analysis of repeated measures in psychiatric research. *Archive of General Psychiatry*. **47**, 770–772.

Elston, R.C. and Grizzle, J.E. (1962). Estimation of time-response curves and their confidence bands. *Biometrics*, **18**, 148–159.

Eriksson, J.G., Forsen, T.J., Osmond, C., Barker, D.J. (2003a). Pathways of infant and childhood growth that lead to type 2 diabetes. *Diabetes Care*. **26**, 3006–3010.

Eriksson, J.G., Forsén, T., Tuomilehto, J., Osmond, C., Barker, D.J. (2003b). Early adiposity rebound in childhood and risk of type 2 diabetes in adult life. *Diabetologia*. **46**, 190–194.

Eriksson, J.G., Forsén, T., Tuomilehto, J., Osmond, C., Barker, D.J.P. (2000). Fetal and childhood growth and hypertension in adult life. *Hypertension*. **36**, 790–794.

Eriksson, J.G., Forsén, T., Tuomilehto, J., Osmond, C., Barker, D.J.P. (2001). Early growth and coronary heart disease in later life: longitudinal study. *British Medical Journal*. **322**, 949–953.

Eriksson, J.G., Forsén, T., Tuomilehto, J., Winter, P.D., Osmond, C., Barker, D.J. (1999). Catch-up growth in childhood and death from coronary heart disease: Longitudinal study. *British Medical Journal*. **318**, 427–431.

Esposito, M., Grusovin, M.G., Papanikolaou, N., Coulthard, P., Worthington, H.V. (2009). Enamel matrix derivative (Emdogain®) for periodontal tissue regeneration in intrabony defects. Cochrane Database of Systematic Reviews 2009, Issue 4. Art. No.: CD003875. DOI: 10.1002/14651858.CD003875.pub3.

Falk, H., Laurell, L., Ravald, N., Teiwik, A., Persson, R. (1997). Guided tissue regeneration therapy of 203 consecutively treated intrabony defects using a bioabsorbable matrix barrier. Clinical and radiographic findings. *Journal of Periodontology*. **68**, 571–581.

Fall, C.H.D., Stein, C.E., Kumaran, K., Cox, V., Osmond, C., Barker, D.J., Hales, C.N. (1998). Size at birth, maternal weight, and type 2 diabetes in South India. *Diabetic Medicine*. **15**, 220–227.

Fisher, R.A. (1915). Frequency distribution of the values of the correlation coefficient in samples from an indefinitely large population. *Biometrika*. **10**, 507–521.

Fitzmaurice, G. (2000). Regression to the mean. *Nutrition*. **16**, 81–82.

Fitzmaurice, G.M., Laird, N.M., Ware, J.H. (2004). *Applied Longitudinal Analysis*. Hoboken, NJ: Wiley.

Forbes, A.B., Carlin, J.B. (2005). Letter to the editor: "Residual change" analysis is not equivalent to analysis of covariance. *Journal of Clinical Epidemiology.* **58**, 540–541.

Forsdahl, A. (1997). Are poor living conditions in childhood and adolescence an important risk factor for arteriosclerotic heart disease? *British Journal of Preventive and Social Medicine.* **31**, 91–95.

Fox, J. (1997). *Applied Regression Analysis, Linear Models, and Related Methods.* Thousand Oaks: Sage.

Frankel, S., Elwood, P., Sweetnam, P. et al. (1996). Birthweight, adult risk factors and incident coronary heart disease: The Caerphilly Study. *Public Health.* **110**, 139–143.

Friedman, L., Wall, M. (2005). Graphical views of suppression and multicollinearity in multiple linear regression. *The American Statistician.* **59**, 127–136.

Friedman, M. (1992). Do old fallacies ever die? *Journal of Economic Literature.* **30**, 2129–2132.

Galton, F. (1886). Regression toward mediocrity in hereditary stature. *Journal of Anthropological Institute of Great Britain and Ireland.* **15**, 246–263.

Garside, R.F. (1963). Letter to the editor: On the analysis of repeated measurements of the same subjects. *Journal of Chronic Diseases.* **16**, 445–447, 448–449.

Geenen, R., van de Vijver, F.J.R. (1993). A simple test of the law of initial value. *Psychophysiology* **30**, 525–530.

Geladi, P. (1988). Notes on the history and nature of partial least squares (PLS) modelling. *Journal of Chemometrics.* **2**, 231–246.

Gilham, W.N. (2009). Cousins: Charles Darwin, Sir Francis Galton and the birth of eugenics. *Significance.* **6**, 132–135.

Gill, J.S., Zezulka, A.V., Beevers, D.G., Davies, P. (1985). Relation between initial blood pressure and its fall with treatment. *Lancet.* **1**, 567–568.

Gillman, M.W., Rich-Edward, J.W. (2000). *Paediatric and Perinatal Epidemiology.* **14**, 192–193.

Gillman, M.W. (2005). Re: "Why evidence for the fetal origins of adult disease might be a statistical artifact: the 'reversal paradox' for the relation between birth weight and blood pressure in later life." (Letter). *American Journal of Epidemiology.* **162**, 292.

Gilthorpe, M.S., Frydenberg, M., Cheng, Y., Baelum, V. (2009). Modelling count data with excessive zeros: The need for class prediction in zero-inflated models and the issue of data generation in choosing between zero-inflated and generic mixture models for dental caries data. *Statistics in Medicine.* **28**, 3539–3553.

Gilthorpe, M.S., Griffiths, G.S., Maddick, I.H., Zamzuri, A.T. (2001). The application of multilevel models to longitudinal dental research data. *Community Dental Health.* **18**, 79–86.

Gilthorpe, M.S., Maddick, I.H., Petrie.A (2000). Introduction to multilevel modelling in dental research. *Community Dent Health.* **17**, 222–6.

Gilthorpe, M.S., Tu, Y.K., Kubzansky, L.D., Goodman, E. (submitted). The importance of accommodating autocorrelation in growth mixture modelling of outcomes in lifecourse epidemiology.

Glantz, S.A., Slinker, B.Y. (2001). *Applied Regression and Analysis of Variance.* New York: McGraw-Hill.

Gluckman, P.D., Hanson, M.A. (2004). The developmental origins of the metabolic syndrome. *Trends in Endocrinology and Metabolism.* **15**, 183–187.

Gluckman, P.D., Hanson, M.A. (2005). *Fetal Matrix: Evolution, Development and Disease.* Cambridge: Cambridge University Press.

Glymour, M.M. (2006). Using causal diagrams to understand common problems. In Oakes, J.M., Kaufman, J.S., editors. *Methods in Social Epidemiology.* San Francesco: Jossey-Bass, pp. 393–428.

Glymour, M.M., Greenland, S. (2008). Causal diagrams. In Rothman, K.J., Greenland, S., and Lash, T., editors. *Modern Epidemiology,* 3rd ed. Raven: Lippincott, pp. 181–210.

Glymour, M.M., Weuve, J., Berkman, L.F., Kawachi, I., Robins, J.M. (2005). When is baseline adjustment useful in analysis of change? An example with education and cognitive change. *American Journal of Epidemiology.* **162**, 267–278.

Gmel, G., Wicki, M., Rehm, J., Heeb, J.L. (2008). Estimating regression to the mean and true effects of an intervention in a four-wave panel study. *Addiction.* **103**, 32–41.

Goldstein, H. (1995). *Multilevel Statistical Models,* 2nd ed. New York: John Wiley & Sons.

Greenland, S., Pearl, J., Robins, J.M. (1999). Causal diagrams for epidemiologic research. *Epidemiology.* **10**, 37–48.

Gumbel, E.J. (1926). Spurious correlation and its significance to physiology. *Journal of American Statistical Association.* **21**, 179–94.

Gunsolley, J.C., Elswick, R.K., Davenport, J.M. (1998). Equivalence and superiority testing in regeneration clinical trials. *Journal of Periodontology.* **69**, 521–527.

Hadi, A.S., Ling, R.F. (1998). Some cautionary notes on the use of principal components regression. *The American Statistician.* **52**, 15–19.

Halverson, J.D., Koehler, R.E. (1981). Gastric bypass: Analysis of weight loss and factors determining success. *Surgery.* **90**, 446–455.

Hand, D.J. (1994). Deconstructing statistical questions. *Journal of the Royal Statistical Society, Series A.* **157**, 317–356.

Hanley, J.A. (2004). "Transmuting" women into men: Galton's family data on human stature. *The American Statistician.* **58**, 237–243.

Harris, R.J. (2004). Clinical evaluation of a composite bone graft with a calcium sulfate barrier. *Journal of Periodontology.* **75**, 685–692.

Hastie, T., Tibshirani, R., Friedman, J. (2009). *The Elements of Statistical Learning: Data Mining, Inference and Prediction,* 2nd ed. New York: Springer.

Hayes, R.J. (1988). Methods for assessing whether change depends on initial value. *Statistics in Medicine.* **7**, 915–927.

Healy, M.J.R. (1981). Some problems in repeated measurements. In Bithell, J.F. and Coppi, R., editors. *Perspectives in Medical Statistics.* London: Academic Press, pp. 151–171.

Heden, G., Wennström, J., Lindhe, J. (1999). Periodontal tissue alterations following Emdogain treatment of periodontal sites with angular bone defects. *Journal of Clinical Periodontology.* **26**, 855–860.

Hennessy, E., Alberman, E. (1998). Intergenerational influences affecting birth outcome. II. Preterm delivery and gestational age in the children of the 1958 British birth cohort. *Paediatric and Perinatal Epidemiology* **1**(12), 61–75.

Hernan, M.A., Hernandez-Diaz, S., Werler, M.M., Mitchell, A.A. (2002). Causal knowledge as a prerequisite for confounding evaluation: An application to birth defects epidemiology. *American Journal of Epidemiology.* **155**, 176–184.

Herr, D.G. (1980). On the history of the use of geometry in the general linear model. *The American Statistician.* **34**, 43–47.

Hjalgrim, L.L., Westergaard, T., Rostgaard, K., Schmiegelow, K., Melbye, M., Hjalgrim, H., Eric, A., Engels, E.A. (2003). Birth weight as a risk factor for child-hood leukemia: A meta-analysis of 18 epidemiologic studies. *American Journal of Epidemiology* **158**, 724–735.

Hoerl, A.E., Kennard, R.W. (1970). Ridge regression: Biased estimation for nonorthog-onal problems. *Technometrics*. **42**, 80–86.

Horst, P. (1941). The role of prediction variables which are independent of the cri-terion. In Horst, P. Ed. *The Prediction of Personal Adjustment*. New York: Social Science Research Council, pp. 431–436.

Hoskuldsson, A. (1988). PLS regression methods. *Journal of Chemometrics*. **2**, 211–228.

Hotelling, H. (1933). Book review: The triumph of mediocrity in business. *Journal of American Statistical Association*. **28**, 463–465.

Hox, J. (2002). *Multilevel Analysis*. Mahwah, NJ: Lawrence Erlbaum Associates.

Huck, S.W., McLean, R.A. (1975). Using a repeated measures ANOVA to analyse the data from a pretest-posttest design: A potential confusing task. *Psychological Bulletin*. **82**, 511–518.

Hujoel, P.P., DeRouen, T.A. (1992). Determination and selection of the optimum number of sites and patients for clinical studies. *Journal of Dental Research*. **71**, 1516–1521.

Huxley, R.R., Neil, A., Collins, R. (2002). Unravelling the fetal origins hypothesis: Is there really an inverse association between birthweight and subsequent blood pressure? *The Lancet*. **360**, 659–665.

Huxley, R.R., Shiell, A.W., Law, C.M. (2000). The role of size at birth and postnatal catch-up growth in determining systolic blood pressure: A systematic review of the literature. *Journal of Hypertension*. **18**, 815–831.

Jackson, J.E. (2003). *A User's Guide to Principal Components*. Hoboken, NJ: Wiley.

Jewell, N.P. (2004). *Statistics for Epidemiology*. London: Chapman & Hall.

Jin, P. (1992). Toward a reconceptualization of the law of initial value. *Psychological Bulletin*. **111**, 176–184.

Joffe, M.M., Rosenbaum, P.R. (1999). Invited commentary: Propensity scores. *American Journal of Epidemiology*. **150**, 327–333.

Jones, B.L., Nagin, D.S., Roeder, K. (2001). A SAS procedure based on mixture models for estimating developmental trajectories. *Sociological Methods and Research*. **29**, 374–393.

Kaldahl, W., Kalkwarf, K., Patil, K., Dyer, J., Bates, R. Jr. (1988). Evaluation of four modalities of periodontal therapy. Mean probing depths, probing attachment level and recession changes. *Journal of Periodontology*. **59**, 783–793.

Keijzer-Veen, M.G., Euser, A.M., van Montfoort, N., Dekker, F.W., Vandenbroucke, J.P., van Houwelingen, H.C. (2005). *Journal of Clinical Epidemiology*. **58**, 1320–1324.

Kirkwood, B., Sterne, J.A.C. (2003). *Medical Statistics* 2nd ed. Oxford: Blackwell.

Kline, R.B. (2005). *Principles and practice of structural equation modeling*. New York: Guildford Press.

Kreuter, F., Muthén, B. (2008). Analyzing criminal trajectory profiles: Bridging multi-level and group-based approaches using growth mixture modelling. *Journal of Quantitative Criminology*. **24**, 1–31.

Kronmal, R.A. (1993). Spurious correlation and the fallacy of the ratio standard revis-ited. *Journal of the Royal Statistical Society Series A*. **156**, 379–392.

Kuh, D., Ben-Shlomo, Y. (2004). *A Life Course Approach to Chronic Disease Epidemiology*. Oxford: Oxford University Press.

Kumar, R., Bandyopadhyay, S., Aggarwal, A.K., Khullar, M. (2004). Relation between birthweight and blood pressure among 7–8 year old rural children in India. *International Journal of Epidemiology*. **33**, 87–91.

Laird, N. (1983). Further comparative analyses of pretest-posttest research design. *The American Statistician*. **37**, 329–330.

Launer, L.J., Hofman, A., Grobbee, D.E. (1993). Relation between birth weight and blood pressure: Longitudinal study of infants and children. *British Medical Journal*. **307**, 1451–1454.

Law, C.M. (2002). Significance of birth weight for the future. *Archive of Diseases in Children, Fetal and Neonatal Edition*. **86**, F7–F8.

Law, C.M., de-Swiet, M., Osmond, C., Fayers, P.M., Barker, D.J., Cruddas, A.M., Fall, C.H. (1993). Initiation of hypertension in utero and its amplification throughout life. *British Medical Journal*. **306**, 240–27.

Leon, D.A., Koupilova, I., Lithell, H.O., Berglund, L., Mohsen, R., Vagero, D., Lithell, U.B., McKeigue, P.M. (1996). Failure to realise growth potential in utero and adult obesity in relation to blood pressure in 50 year old Swedish men. *British Medical Journal*. **312**, 401–406.

Leon, D.A., Lithell, H.O., Vågerö, D., Koupilova, I., Mohsen, R., Berglund, L., Lithell, U.B., McKeigue, P.M. (1998). Reduced fetal growth rate and increased risk of death from ischaemic heart disease: Cohort study of 15000 Swedish men and women born 1915–29. *British Medical Journal*. **317**, 241–245.

Levitt, N.S., Krisella, S., De Wet, T., Morrell, C., Edwards, R., Ellison, G.T., Cameron, N. (1999). An inverse relation between blood pressure and birth weight among 5 year old children from Soweto, South Africa. *Journal of Epidemiology and Community Health*. **53**, 264–268.

Lewis, J.W., Escobar, L.A. (1986). Suppression and enhancement in bivariate regression. *The Statistician*. **35**, 17–26.

Ley, D., Stale, H., Marsal, K. (1997). Aortic vessel wall characteristics and blood pressure in children with intrauterine growth retardation and abnormal foetal aortic blood flow. *Acta Paediatrica*. **86**, 299–305.

Lindhe, J., Westfelt, E., Nyman, S., Socransky, S.S., Haffajee, A.D. (1984). Long-term effect of surgical/non-surgical treatment of periodontal disease. *Journal of Clinical Periodontology*. **11**, 448–458.

Lindley, D.V. (2001). Linear hypothesis: Fallacies and interpretive problems (Simpson's Paradox). In *International Encyclopaedia of the Social and Behavioural Sciences*, pp. 8881–8884.

Lipkin, E.W., Ott, S.M., Chestnut III, C.H., Chait, A. (1988). Mineral loss in the parenteral nutrition patients. *American Journal of Clinical Nutrition*. **47**, 515–523.

Loehlin, J.C. (2004). *Latent Variable Models*, 4th ed. Mahwah, New Jersey: Lawrence Erlbaum Associates.

Loos, B., Nylund, K., Claffey, N., Egelberg, J. (1989). Clinical effects of root debridement in molar and non-molar teeth. *Journal of Clinical Periodontology*. **16**, 498–504.

Lord, F.M. (1967). A paradox in the interpretation of group comparisons. *Psychological Bulletin*. **68**, 304–305.

Lord, F.M. (1969). Statistical adjustments when comparing preexisting groups. *Psychological Bulletin*. **72**, 336–337.

Lucas, A., Fewtrell, M.S., Cole, T.J. (1999). Fetal origins of adult disease—the hypothesis revisited. *British Medical Journal*. **319**, 245–249.

Lucas, A., Morley, R., Cole, T.J. (1998). Randomised trial of early diet in preterm babies and later intelligence quotient. *British Medical Journal.* **317**, 1481–1487.

Luellen, J.K., Shadish, W.R., Clark, M.H. (2005). Propensity scores: An introduction and experimental test. *Evaluation Review.* **29**, 530–558.

Lynn, H.S. (2003). Suppression and confounding in action. *American Statistician.* **57**, 58–61.

MacCallum, R.C., Zhang, S., Preacher, K.J., Rucker, D.D. (2002). On the practice of dichotomisation of quantitative variables. *Psychological Methods.* **7**, 19–40.

MacKinnon, D.P. (2008). *Introduction to Statistical Mediation Analysis.* Mahwah, NJ: Erlbaum.

MacKinnon, D.P., Krull, J.L., Lockwood, C.M. (2000). Equivalence of the mediation, confounding and suppression effect. *Prevention Science.* **4**, 173–181.

Maddala, G.S. (2001). *Introduction to Econometrics,* 3rd ed. Chichester: John Wiley & Sons.

Maloney, C.J., Rastogi, S.C. (1970). Significance test for Grubb's estimators. *Biometrics.* **26**, 671–676.

Mandel, J. (1982). Using the singular value decomposition in regression analysis. *The American Statisticians.* **36**, 15–24.

McMillen, I.C., Robinson, J.S. (2005). Developmental origins of the metabolic syndrome: Prediction, plasticity, and programming. *Physiological Review.* **85**, 571–633.

McNamee, R. (2003). Confounding and confounders. *Occupational and Environmental Medicine.* **60**, 227–234.

Michels, K.B., Trichopoulos, D., Robins, J.M., Rosner, B.A., Manson, J.E., Hunter, D.J., Colditz, G.A., Hankinson, S.E., Speizer, F.E., Willett, W.C. (1996). Birthweight as a risk factor for breast cancer. *The Lancet.* **348**, 1542–1546.

Miles, J., Shelvin, M. (2001). *Applying Regression and Correlation.* London: Sage.

Miller, A. (2002). *Subset selection in regression.* Boca Raton: Chapman & Hall/CRC.

Moher, D., Schulz, K.F., Altman, D.G. (2001). The CONSORT statement: Revised recommendations for improving the quality of reports of parallel group randomized trials. *BMC Medical Research Methodology.* **1**, 2.

Mohr, L.B. (2000). Regression artifacts and other customs of dubious desert. *Evaluation and Program Planning.* **23**, 397–409.

Montenegro, R., Needleman, I.G., Moles, D.R., Tonetti, M. (2002). Quality of RCTs in periodontology—A systematic review. *Journal of Dental Research.* **81**, 866–870.

Moreno, L.F., Stratton, H.H., Newell, J.C., Feustel, P.J. (1986). Mathematical coupling of data: Correction of a common error for linear calculations. *Journal of Applied Physiology.* **60**, 335–343.

Morgan, W. (1939). A test for the significance of the differences between two variances in a sample from a normal bivariate distribution. *Biometrika.* **31**, 13–19.

Morton, V., Torgerson, D.J. (2003). Effect of regression to the mean on decision making in health care. *British Medical Journal.* **326**, 1083–1084.

Moyé, L.A. (2000). *Statistical Reasoning in Medicine: The Intuitive P-Value Primer.* New York: Springer

Muthén, B., Muthén, L.K. (2000). Integrating person-centered and variable-centered analyses: Growth mixture modeling with latent trajectory classes. *Alcoholism: Clinical and Experimental Research.* **24**, 882–891.

Myles, P.S., Gin, T. (2000). *Statistical Methods for Anaethesia and Intensive Care.* Oxford: Butterworth and Heinemann.

Myrtek, M., Foerster, F. (1986). The law of initial value: A rare exception. *Biological Psychology.* **22**, 227–237.

Neyman, J. (1952). *Lectures and Conferences on Mathematical Statistics and Probability.* Washington, DC: U.S. Department of Agriculture.

Nilsson, P.M., Ostergren, P.O., Nyberg, P., Soderstrom, M., Allebeck, P. (1997). Low birth weight is associated with elevated systolic blood pressure in adolescence: A prospective study of a birth cohort of 149378 Swedish boys. *Journal of Hypertension.* **15**, 1627–31.

Oldham, P.D. (1962). A note on the analysis of repeated measurements of the same subjects. *Journal of Chronic Diseases.* **15**, 969–977.

Oldham, P.D. (1963). Letter to the editor. *Journal of Chronic Diseases.* **16**, 447–448, 449–450.

Ong, K.K., Ahmed, M.L., Emmett, P.M., Preece, M.A., Dunger, D.B. (2000). Association between postnatal catch-up growth and obesity in childhood: Prospective cohort study. *British Medical Journal.* **320**, 967–971.

Paneth, N., Ahmed, F., Stein, A.D. (1996). Early nutritional origins of hypertension: A hypothesis still lacking support. *Journal of Hypertension.* **14**, S121–S129.

Paneth, N., Susser, M. (1995). Early origin of coronary heart disease (the "Barker hypothesis"). *British Medical Journal.* **310**, 411–412.

Pearl, J. (2000). *Causality.* Cambridge: Cambridge University Press.

Pearson, K. (1897). On a form of spurious correlation which may arise when indices are used in the measurement of organs. *Proceedings of the Royal Society in London.* **60**, 489–498.

Pearson, K., Lee, A., Bramley-Moore, L. (1899). Mathematical contributions to the theory of evolution: VI—Genetic (reproductive) selection: Inheritance of fertility in man, and of fecundity in thoroughbred racehorses. *Philosophical Transactions of the Royal Society of London, Series A.* **192**, 257–330.

Pedhazur, E.J. (1997). *Multiple Regression in Behavioral Research: Explanation and Prediction.* Fort Worth: Harcourt.

Phatak, A., de Jong, S. (1997). The geometry of partial least squares. *Journal of Chemometrics.* **11**, 311–338.

Phatak, A., Reilly, P.M., Penlidis, A. (1992). The geometry of 2-block partial least squares regression *Communications in Statistics—Theory and Methods.* **21**, 1517–1553.

Pihlstrom, B.L., Ortiz-Campos, C., McHugh, R.B. (1981). A randomized four-year study of periodontal therapy. *Journal of Periodontology.* **52**, 227–242.

Pitman, E. (1939). A note on normal correlation. *Biometrika.* **31**, 9–12.

Pontoriero, R., Wennström, J., Lindhe, J. (1999). The use of barrier membranes and enamel matrix proteins in the treatment of angular bone defects. *Journal of Clinical Periodontology.* **26**, 833–840.

Power, C., Li, L., Manor, O., Davey Smith, G. (2003). Combination of low birth weight and high adult body mass index: At what age is it established and what are its determinants? *Journal of Epidemiology and Community Health.* **57**, 969–973.

Rasmussen, K.M. (2001). The "fetal origins" hypothesis: Challenges and opportunities for maternal and child nutrition. *Annual Review of Nutrition.* **21**, 73–95.

Reichardt, C.S. (2000). Regression facts and artifacts. *Evaluation and Program Planning.* **23**, 411–414.

Rich-Edwards, J.W., Colditz, G.A., Stampfer, M.J., Willett, W.C., Gillman, M.W., Hennekens, C.H., Speizer, F.E., Manson, J.E. (1999). Birthweight and the risk of type 2 diabetes mellitus in adult women. *Annals of Internal Medicine.* **130**, 278–284.

Rich-Edwards, J.W., Stampfer, M.J., Manson, J.E., Rosner, B., Hankinson, S.E., Colditz, G.A., Willett, W.C., Hennekens, C.H. (1997). Birth weight and risk of cardiovascular disease in a cohort of women followed up since 1976. *British Medical Journal.* **315**, 369–400.

Rothman, K. (2002). *Epidemiology: An Introduction.* New York: Oxford University Press.

Rubin, D.B. (1997). Estimating causal effects from large data sets using propensity scores. *Annals of Internal Medicine.* **127**, 757–763.

Saville, D.J., Wood, G.R. (1991). *Statistical Methods: The Geometric Approach.* New York: Springer.

Saville, D.J., Wood, G.R. (1996). *Statistical Methods: A Geometric Primer.* New York: Springer.

Schluchter, M.D. (2003). Publication bias and heterogeneity in the relationship between systolic blood pressure, birth weight, and catch-up growth—A meta-analysis. *Journal of Hypertension.* **21**, 273–9.

Selvin, S. (1994). *Practical Biostatistical Methods.* Pacific Grove, CA: Duxbury.

Senn, S.J. (1994). Letter to the editor: Importance of trends in the interpretation of an overall odds ratio in the meta-analysis of clinical trials. *Statistics in Medicine.* **13**, 293–295.

Senn, S.J. (1997). *Statistical Issues in Drug Development.* Chichester: Wiley.

Senn, S.J. (2003). *Dicing with Death.* Cambridge: Cambridge University Press.

Senn, S.J. (2006). *Statistical Issues in Drug Development.* Chichester: Wiley.

Sharp, S.J., Thompson, S.G., Altman, D.G. (1996). The relation between treatment benefit and underlying risk in meta-analysis. *British Medical Journal.* **313**, 735–738.

Simon, H.A. (1954). Spurious correlation: A causal interpretation. *Journal of the American Statistical Association.* **49**, 467–492.

Simpson, E.H. (1951). The interpretation of interaction in contingency tables. *Journal of the Royal Statistical Society, Series B.* **13**, 238–241.

Singhal, A., Cole, T.J., Fewtrell, M., Kennedy, K., Stephenson, T., Elias-Jones, A., Lucas, A. (2007). Promotion of faster weight gain in infants born small for gestational age: Is there an adverse effect on later blood pressure? *Circulation.* **115**, 213–220.

Singhal, A., Cole, T.J., Lucas, A. (2001). Early nutrition in preterm infants and later blood pressure: Two cohorts after randomised trials. *Lancet.* **357**, 413–419.

Skidmore, P.M., Hardy, R.J., Kuh, D.J., Langenberg, C., Wadsworth, M.E. (2007). Life course body size and lipid levels at 53 years in a British birth cohort. *Journal of Epidemiology and Community Health.* **61**, 215–220.

Slinker, B.Y., Glantz, S.A. (1985). Multiple regression for physiological data analysis: The problem of multicollinearity. *American Journal of Physiology.* **249**, R1–R12.

Stein, A.D., Thompson, A.M., Waters, A. (2005). Childhood growth and chronic disease: Evidence from countries undergoing the nutrition transition. *Maternal and Child Nutrition.* **1**, 177–184.

Stettler, N., Zemel, B.S., Kumanyika, S., Stallings, V.A. (2002). Infant weight gain and childhood overweight status in a multicenter, cohort study. *Pediatrics.* **109**, 194–199.

Stevens, J.P. (2002). *Applied Multivariate Statistics for the Social Sciences,* 4th ed. New Jersey: Lawrence Erlbaum Associates.

Stigler, S.M. (1997). Regression towards the mean, historically considered. *Statistical Methods in Medical Research.* **6**, 103–114.

Stigler, S.M. (1999). *Statistics on the Table.* Cambridge, Massachusetts: Harvard University Press.

Stocks, N.P., Davey Smith, G. (1999). Blood pressure and birthweight in first year university students aged 18–25. *Public Health.* **113**, 273–277.

Stone, M., Brooks, R.J. (1990). Continuum regression: Cross-validated sequentially constructed prediction embracing ordinary least squares, partial least squares and principal components regression. *Journal of the Royal Statistical Society, Series B.* **52**, 237–269.

Stratton, H.H., Feustel, P.J., Newell, J.C. (1987). Regression of calculated variables in the presence of shared measurement error. *Journal of Applied Physiology.* **62**, 2083–2093.

Szklo, M., Nieto, F.J. (2004). *Epidemiology: Beyond the Basics.* Sudbury, Massachusetts: Jones and Bartlett.

Taylor, C.E., Jones, H., Zaregarizi, M., Cable, N.T., George, K.P., Atkinson, G. (2010). Blood pressure status and post-exercise hypotension: An example of a spurious correlation in hypertension research? *Journal of Human Hypertension.* **24**, 585–592.

Taylor, J.M.G., Yu, M. (2002) Bias and efficiency loss due to categorizing an explanatory variable. *Journal of Multivariate Analysis.* **83**, 248–263.

Thompson, S.G., Smith, T.C., Sharp, S.J. (1997). Investigating underlying risk as a source of heterogeneity in meta-analysis. *Statistics in Medicine.* **16**, 2741–2758.

Tu, Y.K. (2005). Statistical issues in medical and dental epidemiology: The problems of mathematical coupling, regression to the mean, collinearity, reversal paradox, and interaction. PhD thesis. University of Leeds, Leeds, UK.

Tu, Y.K., Baelum, V., Gilthorpe, M.S. (2005a). The relationship between baseline value and its change: Problems in categorization and the proposal of a new method. *European Journal of Oral Sciences.* **113**, 279–288.

Tu, Y.K., Baelum, V., Gilthorpe, M.S. (2008a). A structural equation modelling approach to the analysis of change. *European Journal of Oral Science.* **116**, 291–296.

Tu, Y.K., Blance, A., Clerehugh, V., Gilthorpe, M.S. (2005b). Statistical power for analyses of changes in randomized controlled trials. *Journal of Dental Research.* **84**, 283–287.

Tu, Y.K., Clerehugh, V., Gilthorpe, M.S. (2004a). Ratio variables in regression analysis can give rise to spurious results: Illustration from two studies in periodontology. *Journal of Dentistry.* **32**, 143–151.

Tu, Y.K., D'Aiuto, F., Baelum, V., Gilthorpe, M.S. (2009a). An introduction to latent growth curve modelling for longitudinal continuous data in dental research. *European Journal of Oral Sciences.* **117**, 343–350.

Tu, Y.K., Ellison, G.T.H., Gilthorpe, M.S. (2006a). Growth, current size and the role of the 'reversal paradox' in the foetal origins of adult disease: An illustration using vector geometry. *Epidemiologic Perspectives and Innovations.* **3**, 9.

Tu, Y.K., Gilthorpe, M.S. (2007). Revisiting the relation between change and initial value: A review and evaluation. *Statistics in Medicine.* **26**, 443–457.

Tu, Y.K., Gilthorpe, M.S., D'Aiuto, F., Woolston, A., Clerehugh, V. (2009b). Partial least squares path modelling for relations between baseline factors and treatment outcomes in periodontal regeneration. *Journal of Clinical Periodontology.* **36**, 984–995.

Tu, Y.K., Gilthorpe, M.S., Ellison, G.T.H. (2006b). What is the effect of adjusting for more than one measure of current body size on the relation between birthweight and blood pressure? *Journal of Human Hypertension.* **20**, 646–657.

Tu, Y.K., Gilthorpe, M.S., Griffiths, G.S. (2002). Is reduction of pocket probing depth correlated with the baseline value or is it 'mathematical coupling'? *Journal of Dental Research.* **81**, 722–726.

Tu, Y.K., Gunnell, D., Gilthorpe, M.S. (2008b). Simpson's paradox, Lord's paradox, and suppression effects are the same phenomenon—The reversal paradox. *Emerging Theme in Epidemiology.* **5**, 2.

Tu Y.K., Kellett M, Clerehugh V., Gilthorpe M.S. (2005c) Problems of correlations between explanatory variables in multiple regression analyses in the dental literature. *British Dental Journal.* **199**, 457–461.

Tu, Y.K., Law, G.R. (2010). Re-examining the associations between family backgrounds and children's cognitive developments in early ages. *Early Child Development and Care.* **180**, 1243–1252.

Tu, Y.K., Maddick, I.H., Griffiths, G.S., Gilthorpe, M.S. (2004b). Mathematical coupling can undermine the statistical assessment of clinical research: Illustration from the treatment of guided tissue regeneration. *Journal of Dentistry.* **32**, 133–142.

Tu, Y.K., Manda, S.O.M., Ellison, G.T.H., Gilthorpe, M.S. (2007). Revisiting the interaction between birth weight and current body size in the foetal origins of adult disease. *European Journal of Epidemiology.* **22**, 565–575.

Tu, Y.K., Nelson-Moon, Z., Gilthorpe, M.S. (2006c). Misuses of correlation and regression analyses in orthodontic research: The problem of mathematical coupling. *American Journal of Orthodontics and Dentofacial Orthopedics.* **130**, 62–68.

Tu, Y.K., West, R., Ellison, G.T.H., Gilthorpe, M. (2005d). Why evidence of fetal origins of adult diseases can be statistical artifact: The reversal paradox examined for hypertension. *American Journal of Epidemiology.* **161**, 27–32.

Tu, Y.K., Woolston, A., Baxter, P.D., Gilthorpe, M.S. (2010). Accessing the impact of body size in childhood and adolescence on blood pressure: An application of partial least squares regression. *Epidemiology,* **21**, 440–448.

Twisk, J., Proper, K. (2004). Evaluation of the results of a randomised controlled trial: How to define changes between baseline and follow-up. *Journal of Clinical Epidemiology.* **57**, 223–228.

Twisk, J.W.R. (2006). *Applied Multilevel Analysis.* Cambridge: Cambridge University Press.

Van Houwelingen, H., Senn, S.J. (1999). Letter to the editor. *Statistics in Medicine.* **18**, 110–113.

Vandenbroucke, J.P. (2002). The history of confounding. *Social and Preventive Medicine.* **47**, 216–24.

Venables, W.N., Ripley, B.D. (2002). *Modern Applied Statistics with S.* New York: Springer.

Vickers, A.J., Altman, D.G. (2001) Analysing controlled trials with baseline and follow up measurements. *British Medical Journal.* **323**, 1123.

Vickers, A.J. (2001). The use of percentage changes from baseline as an outcome in a controlled trial is statistically inefficient: A simulation study. *BMC Medical Research Methodology.* **1**, 6.

Wainer, H. (1991). Adjusting for Differential Base Rates: Lord's Paradox Again. *Psychological Bulletin.* **109**, 147–151.

Wakeling, I.N., Morris, J.J. (1993). A test of significance for partial least squares regression. *Journal of Chemometrics.* **7**, 291–304.

Walker, S.P., Gaskin, P., Powell, C.A., Bennett, F.I., Forrester, T.E., Grantham-McGregor, S. (2001). The effects of birth weight and postnatal linear growth retardation on blood pressure at age 11–12 years. *Journal of Epidemiology and Community Health.* **55**, 394–398.

Wartenberg, D., Northridge, M. (1994). Letter to the editor: Reply. *American Journal of Epidemiology*. **139**, 443–444.

Weinberg, C. (2005). Barker meets Simpson. *American Journal of Epidemiology*. **161**, 33–35.

Weinberg, C.R. (1993). Toward a clearer definition of confounding. *American Journal of Epidemiology*. **137**, 1–8.

Wen, C.P., Tsai, M.K., Chung, W.S., Hsu, H.L., Chang, Y.C., Chan, H.T., Chiang, P.H., Cheng, T.Y., Tsai, S.P. (2010). Cancer risks from betel quid chewing beyond oral cancer: A multiple-site carcinogen when acting with smoking. *Cancer Causes and Control*. **21**, 1427–35.

Whincup, P.H., Bredow, M., Payne, F., Sadler, S., Golding, J. (1999). Size at birth and blood pressure at 3 years of age: The Avon Longitudinal Study of Pregnancy and Childhood (ALSPAC). *American Journal of Epidemiology*. **149**, 730–39.

Wickens, T.D. (1995). *The Geometry of Multivariate Statistic*. Hillsdale, NJ: Lawrence Erlbaum Associates.

Wilcox, A.J. (2001). On the importance-and the unimportance-of birthweight. *International Journal of Epidemiology*. **30**, 1233–1241.

Williams, S., Poulton, R. (2002). Birth size, growth, and blood pressure between the ages of 7 and 26 years: Failure to support the foetal origins hypothesis. *American Journal of Epidemiology*. **155**, 849–852.

Woelk, G., Emanuel, I., Weiss, N.S., Psaty, B.M. (1998). Birthweight and blood pressure among children in Harare, Zimbabwe. *Archive of Diseases in Children, Fetal and Neonatal Edition*. **79**, F119–F122.

Wold, H. (1982). Soft modeling: The basic design and some extensions. In Jöreskog, K., Wold, H., editors. *Systems under Indirect Observation*, volume 2. Amsterdam: North Holland.

Wold, S., Sjöström, M., Eriksson, L. (2001). PLS-regression: A basic tool of chemometrics. *Chemometrics and Intelligent Laboratory Systems*. **58**, 109–130.

Wonnacott, T.H., Wonnacott, R.J. (1979). *Econometrics*. New York: Wiley.

Wonnacott, T.H., Wonnacott, R.J. (1981). *Regression: A Second Course in Statistics*. New York: Wiley.

Yiu, V., Buka, S., Zurakowski, D., McCormick, M., Brenner, B., Jabs, K. (1999). Relationship between birthweight and blood pressure in childhood. *American Journal of Kidney Diseases*. **33**, 253–260.

Yuan, W., Basso, O., Sorensen, H.T., Olsen, J. (2002). Fetal growth and hospitalization with asthma during early childhood: A follow-up study in Denmark. *International Journal of Epidemiology*. **31**, 1240–1245.

Yudkin, P.L., Stratton, H.H. (1996). How to deal with regression to the mean in intervention studies. *The Lancet*. **347**, 241–243.

Yule, G.U. (1903). Notes on the theory of association of attributes in statistics. *Biometrika*. **2**, 121–34.

Yule, G.U. (1910). On the interpretation of correlation between indices or ratios. *Journal of the Royal Statistical Society Series A*. **73**, 644–647.

Zhao, L.P., Kolonel, L.N. (1992). Efficiency loss from categorising quantitative exposures into qualitative exposures in case-control studies. *American Journal of Epidemiology*. **136**, 464–474.

Zitzmann, N.U., Rateischak-Plüss, E., Marinello, C. (2003). Treatment of angular bone defects with a composite bone grafting material in combination with a collagen membrane. *Journal of Periodontology*. **74**, 687–694.

Index

Milton Keynes UK
Ingram Content Group UK Ltd.
UKHW040102071024
449327UK00019B/736